To Debbie- Happy Trails!

Stacy Holden

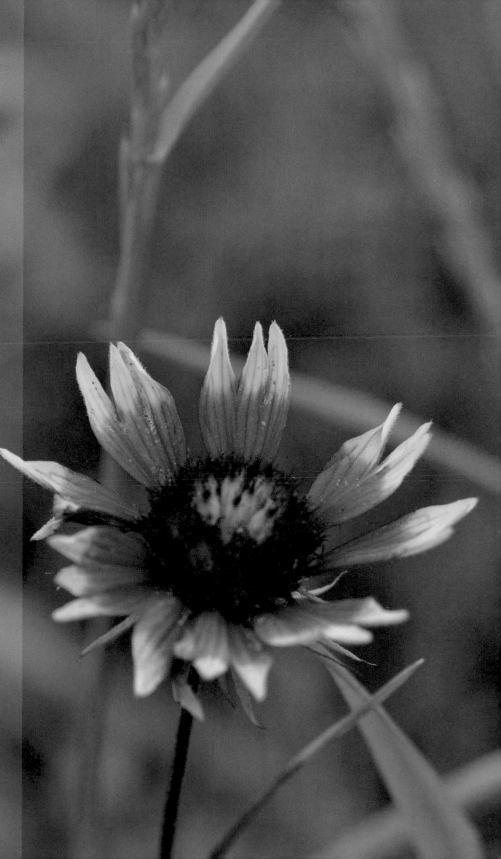

Praise for Stacy Holden & People of Memorial Park

"In her wonderful coffee table book, People of Memorial Park: Stories from Houston's Favorite Trail, *Stacy Holden vividly depicts the wonderful jewel that is the Bayou City's favorite park and the myriad of people who utilize its multitude of resources each day. The uplifting and inspiring stories of redemption and renewal—along with fantastic photography—will inspire readers to tackle and overcome their own hardships."*

—LANCE PHEGLEY, editor, *Texas Runner and Triathlete*

"Memorial Park is my favorite place in all of Houston. In fact, seeing it when I flew into Texas for a job interview in 1991 convinced me to stay. Thank you, Stacy, for recognizing the importance of immortalizing this magical oasis in the heart of the city."

—LISA MALOSKY, CEO, Lisa Malosky Productions;
former sports anchor, KPRC TV2; former cohost, *American Gladiators*

"We are currently implementing a long-range master plan for Memorial Park. In our research to help inform this plan, we have found that people from over 150 zip codes from across the region visit Memorial Park. It is timely and important that a book like this help convey the love that Houstonians have for Memorial Park and the important role that the Park plays in their lives."

—SHELLYE ARNOLD, president and CEO, Memorial Park Conservancy

PEOPLE OF MEMORIAL PARK

PEOPLE OF MEMORIAL PARK

Stories From Houston's Favorite Trail

STACY HOLDEN

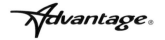

Published by Advantage, Charleston, South Carolina.
Member of Advantage Media Group.

ADVANTAGE is a registered trademark and the Advantage colophon is a trademark of Advantage Media Group, Inc.

Printed in the United States of America.

ISBN: 978-1-59932-806-5
LCCN: 2016953155

Cover design by Katie Biondo.

This publication is designed to provide accurate and authoritative information in regard to the subject matter covered. It is sold with the understanding that the publisher is not engaged in rendering legal, accounting, or other professional services. If legal advice or other expert assistance is required, the services of a competent professional person should be sought.

Advantage Media Group is proud to be a part of the Tree Neutral® program. Tree Neutral offsets the number of trees consumed in the production and printing of this book by taking proactive steps such as planting trees in direct proportion to the number of trees used to print books. To learn more about Tree Neutral, please visit **www.treeneutral.com.**

Advantage Media Group is a publisher of business, self-improvement, and professional development books. We help entrepreneurs, business leaders, and professionals share their Stories, Passion, and Knowledge to help others Learn & Grow. Do you have a manuscript or book idea that you would like us to consider for publishing? Please visit **advantagefamily.com** or call **1.866.775.1696.**

To my family: my parents who introduced me to the Park in 1988; my grandfathers who took me to the Park many times before I was old enough to drive myself; my grandmother and aunt who encouraged me to start writing; my husband and daughters who have patiently walked through the entire process; and my entire extended family who read my WhatsApp updates, prayed for me, voted on titles, and constantly made me feel like they were excited about what I was doing.

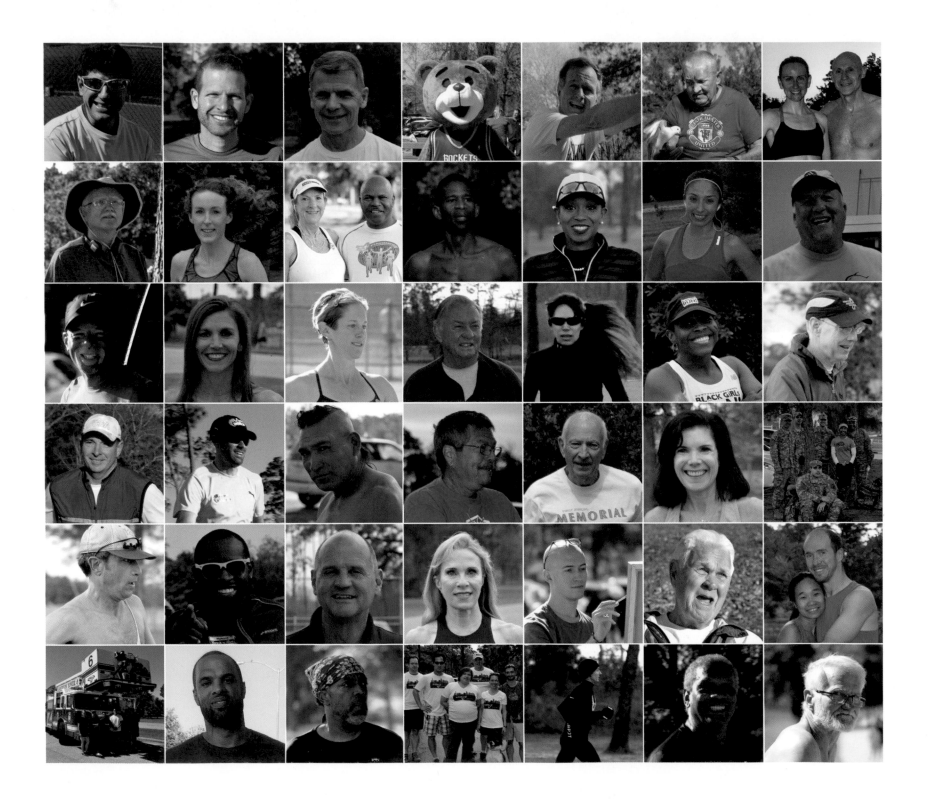

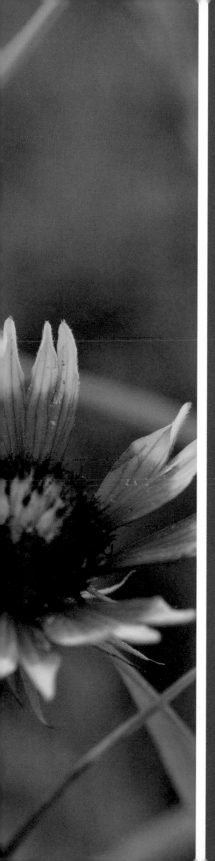
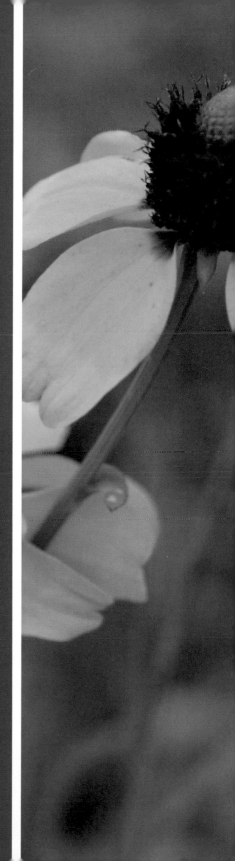

Table of Contents

Stories from the Trail

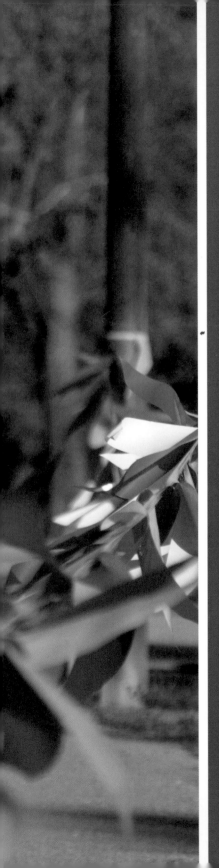

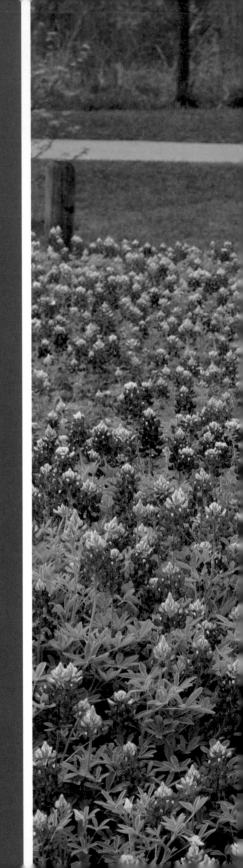

Acknowledgments

I first want to praise Jesus for using me to write this book. As a numbers girl, I am the last person in the world I would have expected to become an author. As the Bible says in 1 Corinthians 2:9, "[N]o mind can conceive what God has in store for those who love Him," and that is certainly true of this entire project.

My husband and mom dutifully read every word I typed and consistently offered their brilliant suggestions on what needed to be changed or improved. There were a couple times when I finished writing a story at midnight and then insisted I needed them to proofread it by 8:00 a.m. the next morning. They never grew weary of my requests, and for that I am truly thankful.

During this time, my girls were beautiful examples of patient, mature young ladies. There were many days when we would go to the Park and plan to only be there for thirty minutes. Inevitably, I would start talking to someone and, an hour later, they would still be quietly waiting for me to finish.

Candice Corley took a majority of the photographs in the book. Her talent can obviously be seen in the final product, but what I appreciated as much as her skill behind the camera was her genuine interest in the people she was photographing. At first I tried to schedule the photo sessions fifteen minutes apart. However, I quickly realized Candice loved the people we were meeting just as much as I did and wanted to spend time talking to them. I finally moved the appointments to every thirty minutes and was constantly reminded of what a delightful, sweet friend she is.

Zachary Nottingham and Wilmer Gaviria also took several pictures that made my stomach flip when I saw them. They both have an innate ability to capture gorgeous images.

The people who are in this book gave me several hours of their time to be interviewed, have their photographs taken, and then review what I had written. Their willingness to help in anything I asked humbles me and makes me eternally grateful.

I could write another entire book called *The Stories Behind the Stories*. There were so many funny things that happened while I was collecting these interviews. More than anything, there were numerous moving parts to tracking down the individuals. A couple of brief examples include the following:

- When I interviewed Catherine Kruppa, she suggested I speak to Wayne and Olya Cohen, who then introduced me to Dan Black, Elvira Hall, and Christy Lan. The Park is a great example of networking. The same is true for Xavi McDuell: she encouraged me to talk to Crystal Hadnott and Ezra Richards. Ezra's sister, Camille, who was home from college on Spring Break, came to Ezra's interview at Black Walnut Café. She suggested I start Facebook and Instagram pages for the book. I told her I did not know how to use Instagram, so they met me at a juice bar the next day and sat for hours helping me set up new accounts.

- As mentioned in his story, Rodney Johnson knows almost everyone at the Park. He tracked down several people to ask if they were okay with me including them. Rodney was the first person I formally interviewed. At the end, right before I turned the voice memo recording off on my phone, he told me he had just been diagnosed with diabetes. I pulled out my insulin pump and said, "Guess what! I also have diabetes!" He was somewhat taken aback by the timing because he had sat in pump training all morning. It was God's perfect timing, but I have also enjoyed becoming friends with someone who truly loves the Park as much as I do.

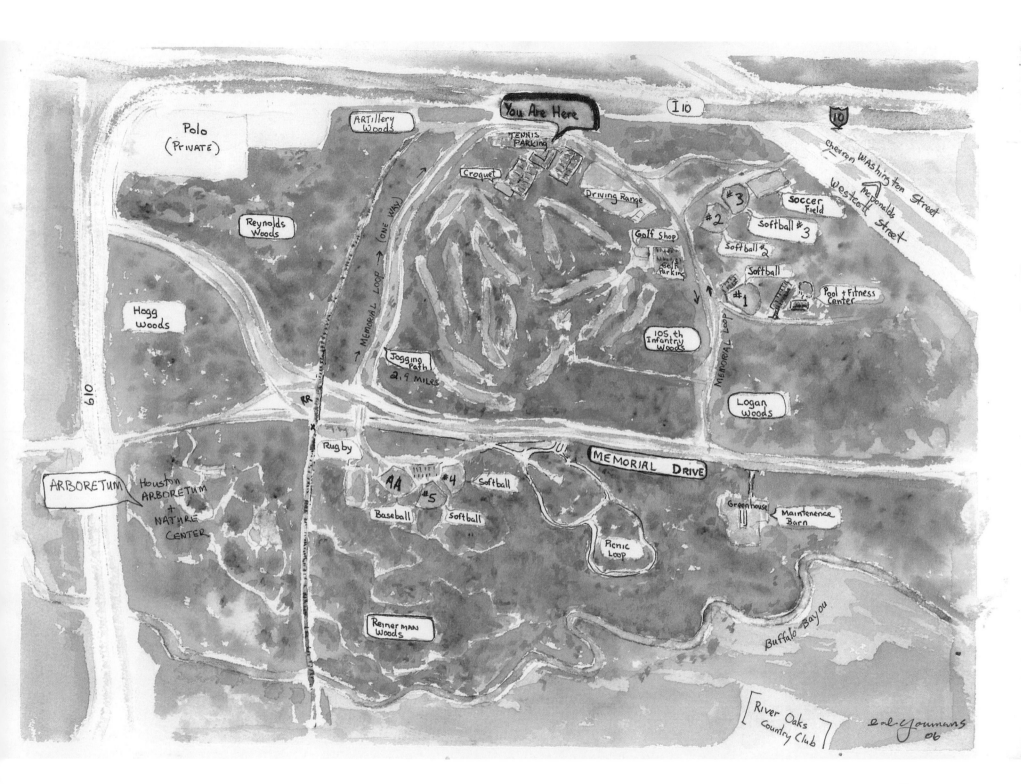

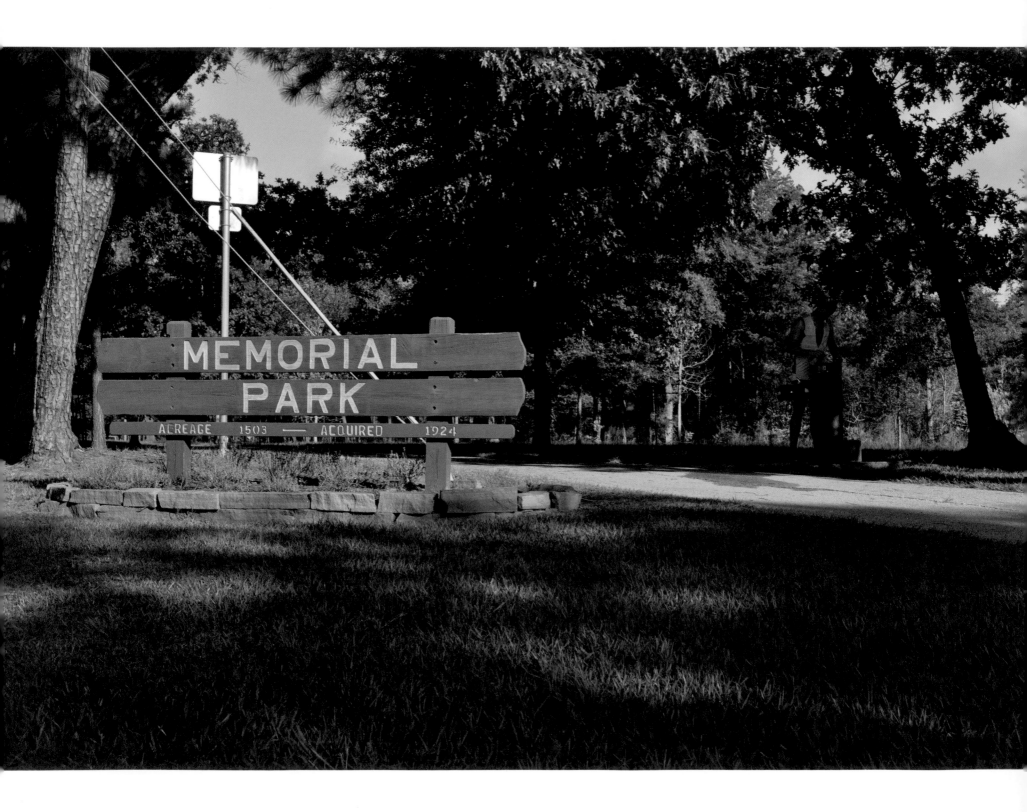

Introduction

In 1917, the United States War Department leased 7,600 acres along Buffalo Bayou to establish a training base named Camp Logan. After World War I, citizens began encouraging the City of Houston to purchase some of that land and turn it into a park in memory of the soldiers. In 1924, the city acquired 1,503 acres and officially established Memorial Park. The 2.9-mile Seymour Lieberman Exer-Trail was built in 1978. It circles a beautiful public golf course and the Tennis Center, which houses a locker room, Smoothie King bar, and eighteen lighted tennis courts. At first the trail was covered in bark mulch, but it was later changed to crushed granite.

In 2011, a drought killed over half the trees in the Park. It was also a dangerous time for users of the trail. There were many places where uncovered roots created tripping hazards, and occasionally branches fell from trees and landed on people and cars. A reforestation plan was established, and more than one hundred thousand trees have been planted in an effort to make the Park the lush area it was before.

Today, an average of ten thousand people use the Park on a daily basis for reasons that include sand volleyball, cycling, golfing, swimming, mountain biking, and playing on the playground. However, a majority of those ten thousand attendees are walking or running on the 2.9-mile trail. Memorial Park is perfectly located within a few miles of downtown Houston, the Galleria, and the Energy Corridor. The Park's proximity to major employers makes it a convenient spot to exercise before or after work.

In 2015, Houston's City Council approved a long-term master plan for the Park. It includes construction of an observation tower, quarter-mile track, boat launch, indoor swimming pool, and many other infrastructure improvements. The project is estimated to cost $300 million and take twenty years to complete. A large portion of the funding is expected to come from private donations.

www.memorialparkconservancy.com

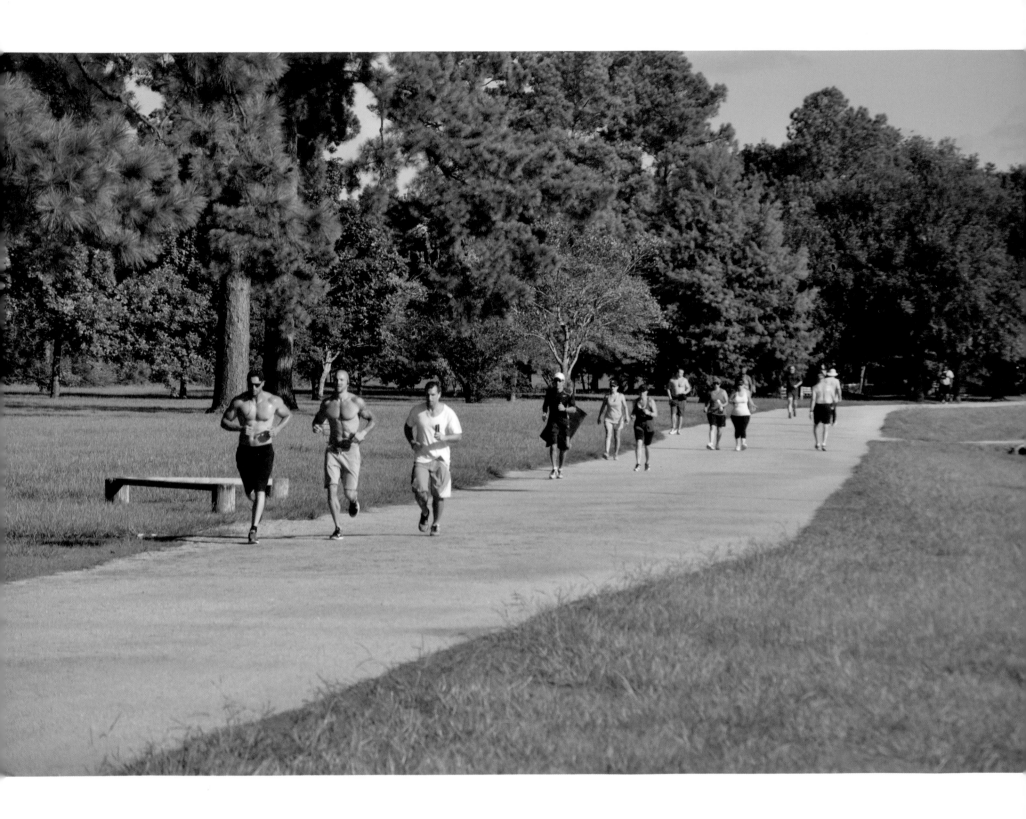

"I Love This Park"

There are several common elements present throughout this book. Although each story is unique, many people share experiences and feelings that unite us all.

- The phrase repeated more than any other was "I love this park." Those who come to Memorial Park on a regular basis find peace, beauty, health, encouragement, and a sense of community that no other gym, neighborhood, or city park offers. It is their home away from home.

- Many people are able to cope with disease and personal tragedy by using the Park as a refuge. It provides a place to channel stress, disappointment, loss, and illness through a positive outlet. Instead of allowing these setbacks to limit or destroy their lives, the strong individuals in this book took ownership of their challenges and decided to seek a better solution.

- The Park offers a social haven, not just a place to exercise. The friendships made there offer a lasting bond that withstands life's trials. Maybe it has something to do with the fact that the people on the trail are side by side and not judging each other; maybe it is because anyone who is working to improve his health and fitness is given a level of respect that the general population does not provide. Regardless of the specific reasons, people come to the Park because of the people.

- After someone has been to the Park a handful of times, he or she becomes familiar with the faces on the trail. Many people discussed how they considered other Park regulars their friends, even though they had never done anything more than wave as they passed. They do not know their names, but still consider them friends.

- A few individuals discussed the strain that a passion for running caused on their marriages. When someone who wants to spend several hours each week working out is married to someone who does not view exercise in the same way, it can cause friction.

- People come to the Park from all over the Houston area. It is common for someone to wake up at 4:00 a.m. and drive for forty-five minutes to get to the Park. Although this means exercising at the Park requires an additional hour and a half of driving over simply running in his or her neighborhood, the Park is worth the time on the road.

- Most of the people in this book were first invited to the Park by a friend. They needed someone to help them figure out what they should do and where they should go. Having a friend who can help to navigate the Park is a tremendous asset.

- There are many different habits people have developed over the years. Some only run in one direction, some listen to music while they run, some chew gum, some always park in the same spot, and some wear the same clothes every day. These rituals are things they have grown accustomed to after years of coming to the Park.

- A majority of the older men who were interviewed for this book freely admit that they enjoy looking at the beautiful women who frequent the Park. These men are not shy about their admiration of the ladies. It is probably safe to assume that most of the younger men also think the Park offers a chance to catch a glimpse of Houston's gorgeous women; the older men are just unashamed to make that proclamation.

Memorial Park, A Park for Everyone

A 2015 survey and user count showed Memorial Park users coming from 170 distinct zip codes in the greater Houston region.

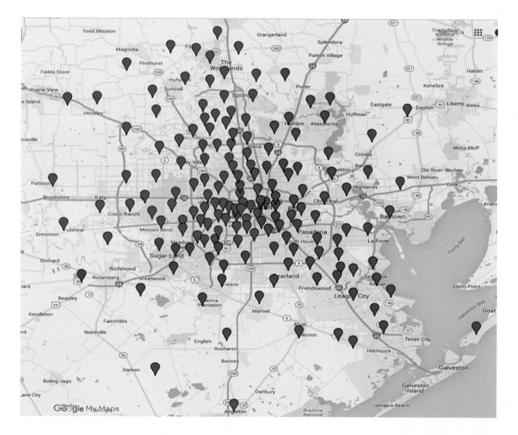

Source: 2015 Memorial Park Master Plan. Based on two-week survey of HARRA (Houston Area Road Runner Association) members who use Memorial Park and two weekends of in-Park survey work.

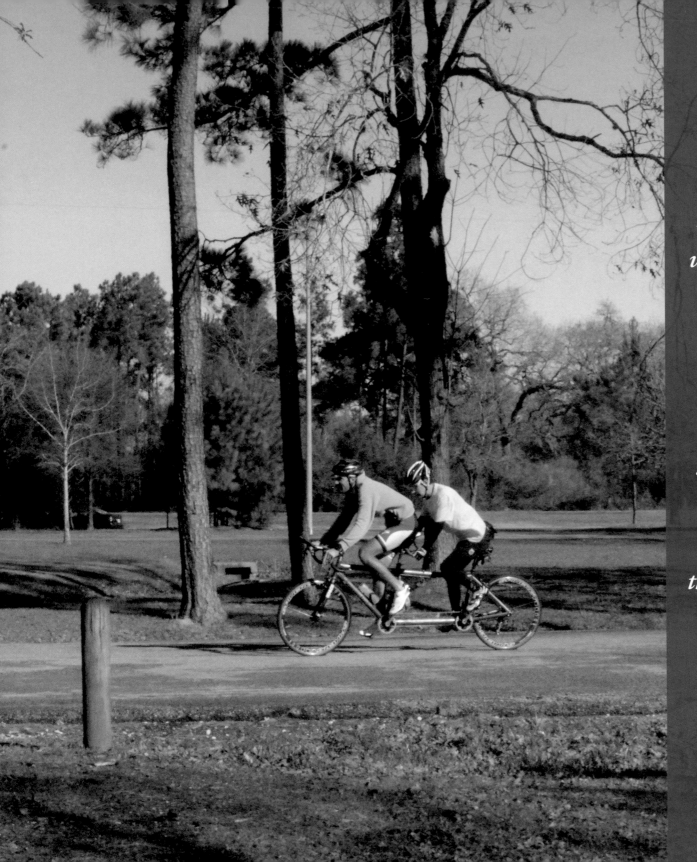

At the age of fifteen, I was sitting in my living room and told my dad that I felt like my eyes were going black. During the last eleven years, I have had over one hundred different guides who also have their own unique stories they could tell about how our paths crossed.

BRANDON ADAME

Shortly after I was born, my pediatrician noticed that my eyes did not dilate when I was placed under light. I went through my first operation to cut slits in my irises when I was four days old, but after each procedure, the openings would close back up, and I would be sent back to the hospital to let the doctors try again. By the time I was six months old, I had been through eight surgeries, but my parents were advised that the effort was worth the hassle because the surgeries would allow me to maintain partial vision. The doctors suggested that even having partial vision was significantly better than not being able to see at all. At the time, my parents and I did not understand the magnitude of what that actually meant.

By the time I was in middle school, I was only able to see small areas of light and distinguish sharp contrasts in color. At the age of fifteen, I was sitting in my living room on a Sunday night and told my dad that I felt like my eyes were going black. The next morning, I headed to school in the same manner I had the previous Friday. The only difference was that over the course of the night, I had become totally blind. My doctors told me that the shape of a person's eyes changes during puberty, but they had no way to predict how that transformation would affect my already limited vision.

When I look back now and think about how my life changed so dramatically from one day to the next, I am reminded of how resilient my family has always been. I have never felt sorry for myself or complained that life is not fair. Instead, I sought to maintain an optimistic outlook and move on, regardless of the difficulties.

I began running in middle school and continued when I went to high school at Texas School for the Blind and Visually Impaired. I was on the track team, and there were wires mounted along the straightaways to guide us. After graduating, my parents wanted to find a way to keep me busy and would often take me to the gym so I could run on a treadmill. My mom's fitness instructor, Mary Lowe, saw me running and came up with an idea. Mary asked the other ladies in the class if they would be interested in training for the upcoming 2006 Houston

Half Marathon. Even though Mary was training for an Ironman triathlon and was one of the fastest women in Houston, she offered to guide me and help me train for the race.

My dad was not at the gym the day Mary came up with her grand plan. When we got home, my mom casually mentioned that we needed to wake up at 5:30 on Saturday morning so we could be at Memorial Park by 6:00 a.m.

When my dad asked why we would ever want to be at Memorial Park that early, my mom proudly announced that we were going to sign up for a half marathon. My dad was not enthusiastic about the situation but knew that refusing to participate was not an option. As I began shuffling around the trail with Mary on that Saturday morning, I had no idea that this was the start of something that would not only change my life but would also allow me to meet hundreds of volunteers who would help me continue exercising.

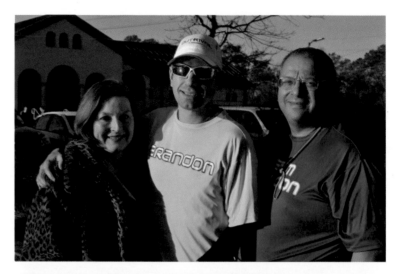

I finished the 2006 race with Mary, and then my parents guided me through the 2007 and 2008 Houston Half Marathons. At first my dad insisted that I carry my cane while I was running, even though I was certain I did not need it. He finally agreed to let me leave it at home because I relied on the person guiding me for every step. A couple months before the 2009 half marathon, Alex Cisne, who is a family friend, contacted my dad and offered to be my guide. He was much faster than my parents, and I enjoyed the freedom to run at a quicker pace.

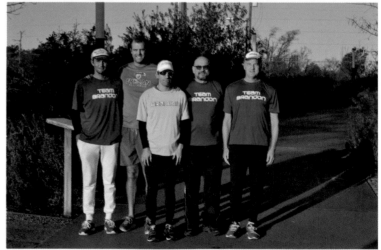

At first, Alex guided me in the same way Mary and my parents had: by keeping one of my hands on his shoulder. However, this was a very inefficient way for us to run. We began experimenting to see if we could figure out a new way to run that would allow both of us to move more naturally. Alex came up with an idea to connect a four-foot rubber tube between each of our arms. The tether gave us the flexibility we were seeking. Over time, we played with the length of the tubing and finally decided that an eighteen-inch tether was best. It allowed both of us to independently swing our arms but still kept me close enough in case Alex needed to grab me.

After my half marathon with Alex, I received several offers from other athletes who were willing to work with me. The next thing I knew, I was being fitted for a tandem bicycle, and I competed in my first triathlon in October 2010. At that time I only knew how to doggie paddle, but a few of my guides also offered to teach me how to swim. Three months later, I started training for the Memorial Hermann Ironman race, which I finished in May 2011. Today I compete in paratriathlons across the United States and have even been able to race in Canada, Mexico, Brazil, Great Britain, and Japan.

Regardless of whether I am training or racing, I enjoy talking to my guides about politics, sports, upcoming races, my life, or anything else that crosses my mind. It does not matter if I am going out for an easy, three-mile run or a fifteen-hour, forty-eight-minute, and forty-second Ironman triathlon—I am never at a loss for words.

During the last eleven years, I have had over one hundred different guides and feel like they all also have their own unique stories they could tell about how our paths crossed. Memorial Park is a convenient location for me to work out because it is centrally located and makes it easy for my guides to meet me. We can ride the bike around the Picnic Loop and then immediately head out for a run. When I run at the Park, I have to rely on my guides to give me instructions for every step I take. They warn me of changes in the surface, direction, or slope of the trail. They also let me know when we need to maneuver around a person, dog, light pole, curb, tree, or anything else that occasionally intersects the path. Most people think the Park is relatively straight and flat with only two sharp turns, but there are actually many bumps, slopes, and meanders in the trail.

I hope that my accomplishments will inspire others to figure out what they need to do to stay active. I am extremely grateful for the individuals who have donated their time and money to support me in my achievements over the last eleven years. Houston's athletic community has been tremendously generous.

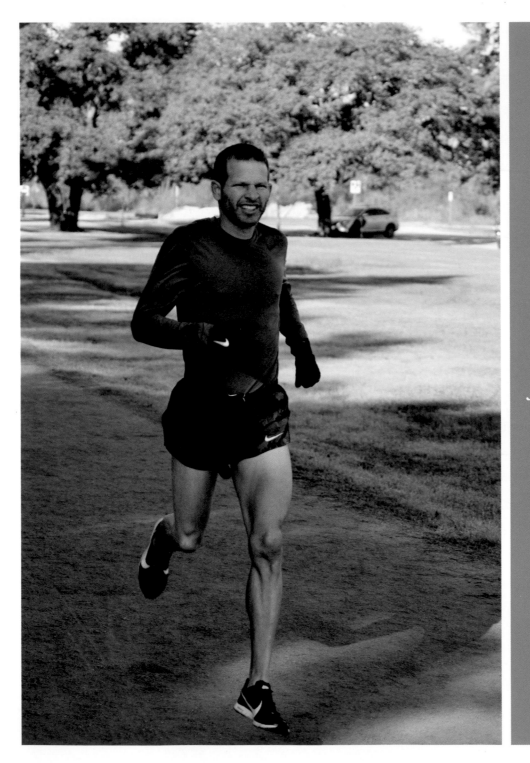

After months of training, we invited several friends and family members to the Memorial Park track to watch the Beer Mile world-record attempt. I finished in five minutes, fifty-one seconds—fourteen seconds faster than the previous world record! We had a huge celebration, which included more beer.

LUIS ARMENTEROS

I grew up in Katy, Texas, and then attended Rice University on a track and cross-country scholarship. After I graduated from college in 1996 and started running on my own, I was a highly undisciplined athlete. Fortunately, I was friends with some of the faster runners in Houston, who welcomed me into their group and introduced me to a very structured, intense way of training. I was exposed to an extremely competitive side of running I had never known, and I began to excel because of their influence.

As marathon running has grown in popularity, there has been a shift toward higher-mileage training. In the late 1990s, though, we focused on speed. Every time our schedule called for an afternoon track workout, I knew I would come home physically and mentally exhausted. We were all very competitive, and our lives focused on running fast. I found Memorial Park to be a very comforting place because it allowed me to piece my shattered ego from the previous workout back together. I regained my confidence and got ready for the next grueling track session.

It was not until 2002, when I started working at a local running store, that I realized there was a different side of running. For the first time, I met people who trained consistently and enjoyed working out but participated for social instead of competitive reasons.

The Park is a great place for people who want to train with their friends or who are looking for a destination for a hard, tempo run. The soft surface of the trail is an added asset. A few years ago, my training partners and I did not care about the type of surface we ran on, but today I know several top runners who, to minimize or prevent injury, refuse to step off the Memorial Park trail unless they are racing.

I also think the Park is a great representation of the changes we have seen in Houston in the last few years. When I started running at the Park after college, there was a small group of dedicated local athletes who worked out there on a regular basis. Today, I see a mix of license plates from across North America. There are individuals who range in age from three to eighty-three. Finally, the Park has some of the fastest runners in the world, along with those who are happy to finish a brisk walk with their beloved dog.

Six years ago, I participated in my first 5K beer run, which started at a bar on Washington Avenue and stopped at four other bars along the way. I anticipated the event would have a party-like atmosphere and be a unique way to combine two of my passions: running and beer.

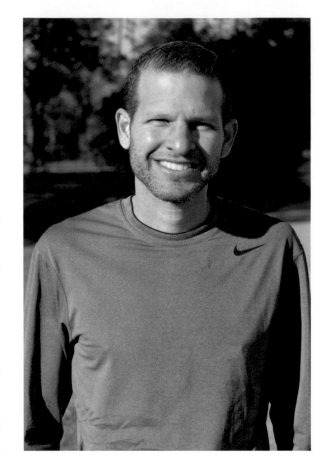

However, another very talented athlete showed up, and he took off running at a five-minute-per-mile pace. Given my competitive nature, I quickly decided that it was time to race. We entered the first bar at the same time, and I guzzled the beer. I looked to my right and saw that he still had half his glass remaining. I took off sprinting and looked back over my shoulder a few times, but he was nowhere in sight. I had just gained twenty seconds on a guy who would have otherwise been right next to me.

A few months later, a friend told me that the Super Masters (forty years old and up) world record for the beer mile was only six minutes, five seconds. In order to complete a beer mile successfully, a competitor drinks a twelve-ounce beer, runs a quarter mile, and then repeats that combination three more times without vomiting. I thought I had a shot at breaking the world record and decided to start training at the Memorial Park quarter-mile track.

My friends supported the endeavor by recording my times and helping figure out how to hand the cans to me. There were a couple days when people who were exercising at the Park would walk up with bewildered faces and ask, "What in the world are you doing with all of this beer? You are running kind of fast . . ."

After months of training, we invited several friends and family members out to watch the world-record attempt. I ended up finishing in five minutes, fifty-one seconds—fourteen seconds faster than the previous world record! We had a huge celebration, which included more beer.

My hope is to still be running competitively when I am in my seventies and beyond. I want to be the old, gray-haired man still fighting to place in my age group on the home stretch of local Houston road races. I guess if I am still running hard in thirty years, I will be relegated to training with the high school girls at Memorial Park. That is a possibility I will just have to learn to live with.

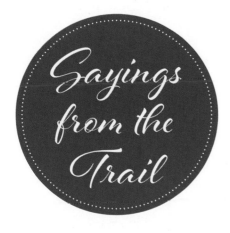

"I didn't recognize you in clothes!"

People come to the Park in workout clothes and athletic shoes. When we see someone in a professional setting, it usually takes a few seconds to realize that the nicely dressed individual is the same sweaty runner we see every day.

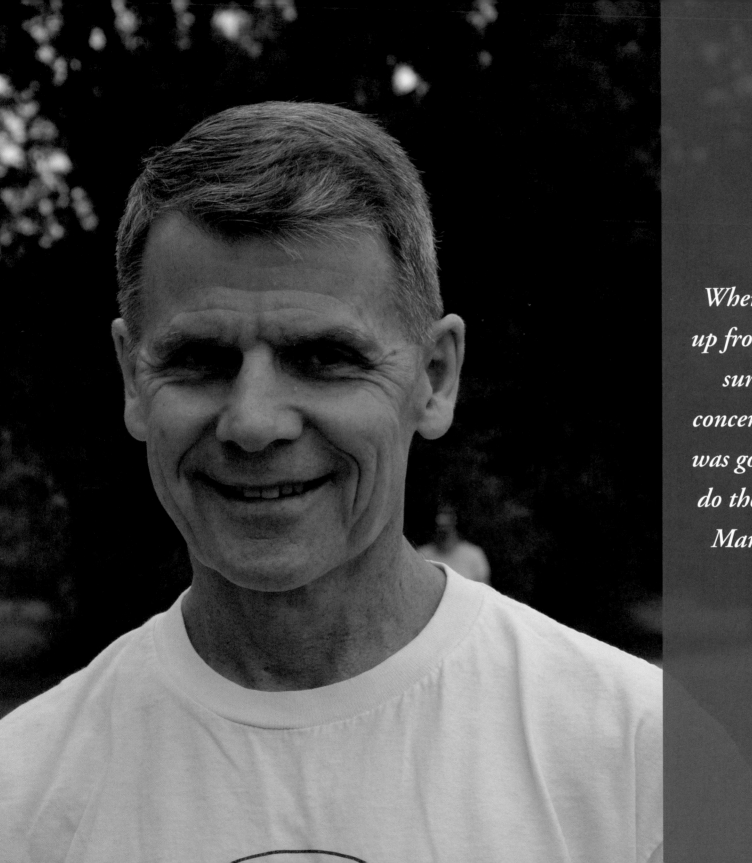

When I finally woke up from my emergency surgery, my only concern was whether I was going to be able to do the New York City Marathon in three months.

DAN BLACK

I taught band for twenty-nine years and started running in my early thirties as a way to relieve stress. Even though I did not know anyone else who ran, it seemed like a smart thing to do. I got hooked real fast.

I went to Memorial Park for the first time in the mid-1990s. Other athletes had spoken fondly of running there, and I finally decided to make the thirty-minute drive to see what they were talking about. Within a couple weeks, I met a wonderful group of people and decided it was worth waking up at 4:00 a.m. so I could join them for my Saturday morning long runs. I liked that the Park was predictable. It was nice to see familiar faces, even if I did not know their names.

After a few years of exercising regularly, I realized that the constant cycle of pushing myself to go farther or faster with each new race was extremely addictive. It was also fun. I finished the Boston Marathon seven times, and in January 2012, I was elated to finally run fast enough to qualify for the New York City Marathon.

Despite the improvements in my running times, I was perplexed by recent episodes of hiccups. During the next few months, the episodes became progressively longer, and I would find myself hiccupping for a couple hours at a time. However, I decided the hiccups were not important, because I was running so well.

I continued to focus on my upcoming New York City Marathon but began to feel fatigued and was frustrated to be reduced to walking. In April 2012, I tried to go for an easy run but felt like I had a total system shutdown only three miles into the workout. By the time I made it home, the hiccups had become volcanic. They lasted for almost nine hours, and I felt like I was having an internal explosion with each breath.

My wife, being the loveable, sweetheart bulldog that she is, insisted I see my doctor immediately. The doctor found I had cancer throughout my esophagus, which was almost completely closed. He also confided to my wife there was no way I would be able to overcome the sickness—and that it would be best not to disclose the discouraging information to me. They agreed to put me on a feeding tube and work to prolong my life, even though the chance of survival was extremely low. I started chemotherapy in May and underwent daily sessions of radiation a few weeks later. I was put on a liquid diet but still raced in two triathlons during the chemo and even won my age group in both of them.

My weight dropped to 130 pounds, but thankfully I responded well to the treatment. A couple of doctors on my medical team said my ability to bounce back was due to the fact I continued to exercise throughout the entire process. I was still bound and determined to run the New York City Marathon in November, but meanwhile, I also needed to have my esophagus rebuilt. I asked my surgeon if it could wait until after the race. Fortunately, she was a runner and understood where I was coming from.

As I was packing my bags for the marathon, Hurricane Sandy hit the East Coast. In spite of the devastation, officials continued to insist the race would go on, so I boarded a plane on Friday morning and flew to New York. Shortly after I checked in at the hotel, I headed out to grab dinner. As I sat in a deli eating the world's worst and most expensive chicken sandwich, I received an e-mail saying the New York City Marathon had been cancelled. A wave of emotions crossed my mind as I thought about all I had been through in the last ten months.

I flew home the next day and decided to go to Memorial Park on Monday. I set up a water station on the hood of my car and started my own personal marathon around the Park. There were no crowds, no announcers, no bridges. More than anything, I just wanted to prove that despite my medical condition, I could finish a marathon faster than the official race cutoff time, which I did.

The following Monday, I entered the hospital for surgery. The recovery was considerably worse than any of the chemo or radiation I had gone through up to that point. I had a feeding tube for a month and felt completely wiped out. In December, after the feeding tube was removed, I resumed my efforts to exercise daily—but not without some setbacks. I tore a muscle in my back while stretching and had to begin physical therapy.

A couple weeks later, I was out jogging and my heart began racing so fast I could not count my pulse rate. It happened again the following week, which was enough to scare me. After going through several tests, I was told I had atrial flutter. Three months after my esophagus was rebuilt, I was lying on the surgeon's table again, this time for my heart. During recovery, I had to lie horizontally. The only problem was the valve that keeps food in the stomach had been removed during my esophagus surgery in November. Everything I ate came right back up.

I was grateful to regain my strength over the next eighteen months, but in August 2014, I was in my bathroom and dropped to the floor with the worst pain I have ever felt in my life. I was in agony. Fortunately my wife was at home, so I pounded on the floor until she finally heard me. I was rushed to the hospital, where the doctor told me I was an hour away from death. The feeding tube from the esophagus surgery had caused internal scarring, and my bowel had wrapped around the scar. That night I lay on the surgeon's table again and had eight feet of bowel removed. I don't remember anything from the two days of recovery because my blood pressure dropped so low that the doctor had to keep me sedated. I was put on watch to see if I would even survive the night.

When I finally woke up, my only concern was whether I was going to be able to do the New York City Marathon in November. My entry from the cancelled race in 2012 was deferred, and I had two years to take advantage of the deferral. Since I was still recovering from the heart surgery in 2013, I decided to wait until 2014 to do the race.

By the end of October, I felt strong enough to run, but when I arrived in New York a week later, I was in a brain fog. Given my dazed state, I was thankful that it was a huge race and there were other runners I could follow. I was finally able to cross the finish line of the New York City Marathon in five hours, thirty-five minutes, but I remember almost nothing about the race. Once I got out of Central Park, it took me three hours to figure out how to hail a cab.

I flew home on Monday and went for a recovery run the next day but could not even finish half a mile. I went to the doctor and found out my iron level was dangerously low. The eight feet of bowel that had been removed was responsible for absorbing iron. Once again, I was admitted into the hospital, this time for a heavy treatment of iron.

I now refer to Memorial Hermann Hospital as my home away from home. I have been forced to admit that I will never be as fast as I was in 2012, but I still swim, bike, and run several times per week and hope to one day get back to racing. I am also still thankful for the predictability of Memorial Park. I am not fast enough to keep up with my former running group, but I like knowing there are several restrooms around the trail; that became important after cancer. I refuse to quit. I will continue to set goals and exercise. There is always hope.

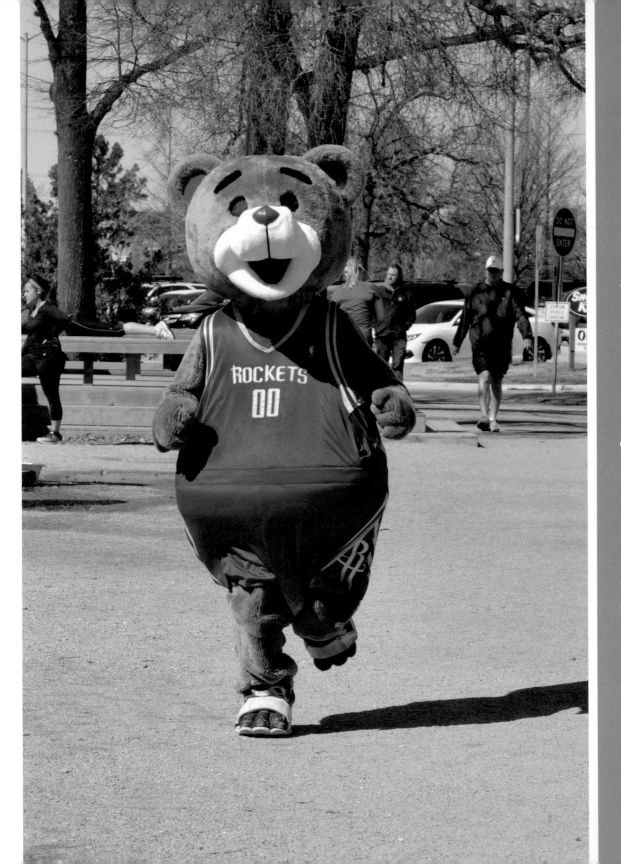

I started running dressed as Clutch "The Rockets Bear" in 2009. I also worked with a costume designer, and over time, we developed a breathable, lightweight uniform that allows me to run without feeling as though I am in a sauna with a bag over my mouth.

ROBERT BOUDWIN, A.K.A. CLUTCH "THE ROCKETS BEAR"

I grew up in Blue Bell, Pennsylvania, and graduated in 1992 from Wissahickon High School. Besides playing soccer, ice hockey, and lacrosse, I was also the school's mascot. Although I was known as the class clown, I generally stayed out of trouble and was just an outgoing kid who had a lot of energy.

During my freshman year at the University of Delaware, I met some cheerleaders who encouraged me to attend the school's mascot audition the following morning. I was thoroughly intimidated, because the enrollment at UD was about three times higher than the population of my entire hometown. However, I decided to show up, and to my surprise, I was chosen to be the mascot!

At that time, each school within the university had its own version of the Fighting Blue Hen, and the mascot's costume consisted of a blue T-shirt and a thin mask. I collaborated with the marketing department to design a more professional uniform and create the mascot's new name: YoUDee. By the end of my sophomore year, the university had officially hired me as a part-time intern in the public-relations department and had awarded me a scholarship for being the mascot.

In 1995, I auditioned and was selected to be Clutch "The Rockets Bear," the new mascot for the Houston Rockets. I eagerly accepted the position and spent the following year creating the character and developing the skills needed to perform my job as Clutch. UD allowed me to take my remaining seven classes at the University of Houston and apply the credits toward the work I had completed before moving to Houston. I was finally able to graduate with a degree in marketing and management from UD in 1997.

Although I ran occasionally to stay in shape for my career, I never considered myself a serious "runner" until my personal life hit a rough patch in 2011. I not only found myself living as a divorced, single father of two young boys but was also forced to admit I had developed terrible eating habits and become overweight. I moved to a neighborhood close to Memorial Park and wanted to find a way to blow off steam. I quickly realized that running provided a means for me to maintain focus and find peace while being able to feel like I had control over a part of my life. In addition to the emotional transformation running afforded, I lost seventy-five pounds in six months! I found solace in knowing the responsibility to work out rested entirely with me. By the end of 2011, I took pride in being able to complete a lap around the Park in less than twenty minutes.

I started running dressed as Clutch "The Rockets Bear" in 2009 to promote the Rockets Run, a 5K that benefits various charities throughout Houston. However, running as a six-foot-eight-inch bear with a ninety-two-inch waist is not easy. Originally, the costume was lined with fur and had thick foam feet that were glued to shoes. I worked with a designer, and over time we developed a breathable, lightweight uniform that allows me to run without feeling as though I am in a sauna with a bag over my mouth.

When the Rockets entered the 2013 NBA playoffs, Clutch announced he would do a 5K at Memorial Park every day to encourage the team and inspire fellow fans. All supporters were invited to accompany him, and on the second day, only one woman showed up. As we began running, she told me that she had finished the Boston Marathon only a couple weeks earlier and was still traumatized by the bombing, which had occurred shortly after she finished the race. She said she had not run since that day but decided to come to the Park with Clutch because it sounded like a fun idea. She needed something that would allow her to run again while taking her mind off the shocking events she had witnessed.

Although Clutch has a warm, gentle smile that never changes, as she was telling me her story, I began crying inside the costume. I was overwhelmed because I helped her heal from the tragedy and run again. Today, any time Clutch or I take part in a fundraiser, that same woman is the first person to donate and has been one of my most generous supporters.

An organization I am passionate about is LifeGift, which facilitates the transfer of organ, eye, and tissue donations to needy recipients throughout Texas. In 2013, my father received a double-lung transplant, and I was astounded by the generosity of the donor and the effort LifeGift contributed to make the procedure possible.

After my father's successful surgery, I decided to establish a group called Team Clutch for the upcoming 2014 Houston Half Marathon. There were twenty runners who joined the team, and we raised $15,000 for LifeGift. I had matching shirts made for our members, but because I was running as Clutch, my shirt had to be size 6XL.

We met at the Park to train for the race and received tremendous support from the people who are there on a regular basis.

I am on the board of directors for LifeGift and have made several public-speaking appearances to spread the organization's message of hope and compassion. Every time I run, I wear a shirt that says, "I Support Organ Donation." I have raised thousands of dollars for LifeGift, and the people who exercise at Memorial Park have contributed about 95 percent of that money. I am grateful for Houston's running community and the generous individuals who appreciate the Park as much as I do!

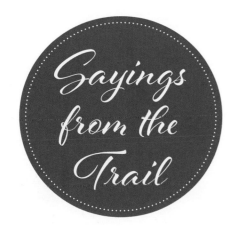

"Let's flip at the pole."

We are going to make a U-turn at the next light pole.

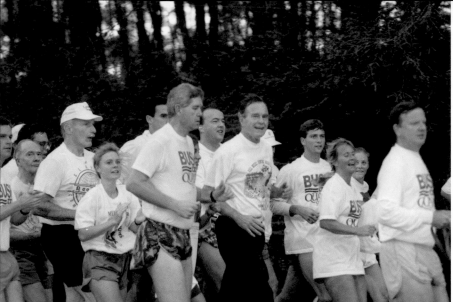

Memorial Park is one of my favorite spots in the world.

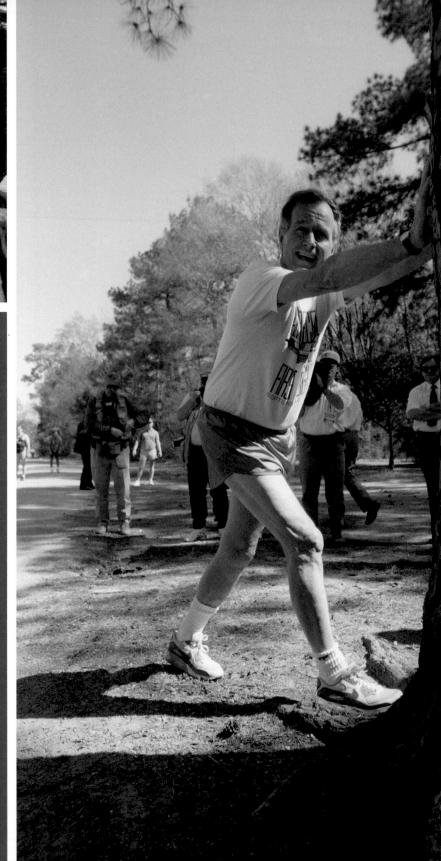

PRESIDENT GEORGE H.W. BUSH

Memorial Park is one of my favorite spots in the world. It has always been a source of great pride for me and, I'm sure, for most Houstonians. The Park is beautiful and offers the citizens of Houston an exceptional venue for many outdoor activities. I've played golf and tennis there, and I spent countless hours running on the Park's paths. I loved every minute; and as a special bonus, I met a lot of wonderful people on those runs.

The Park's history is also a source of pride for me, serving as it did as a World War I army training camp and then being named Memorial Park to honor the memory of soldiers who died in combat during World War I.

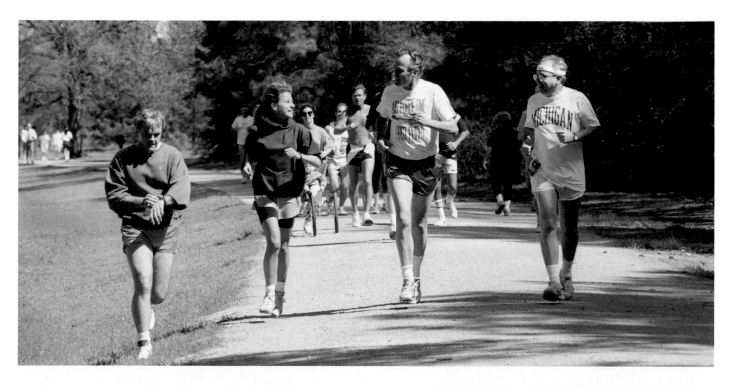

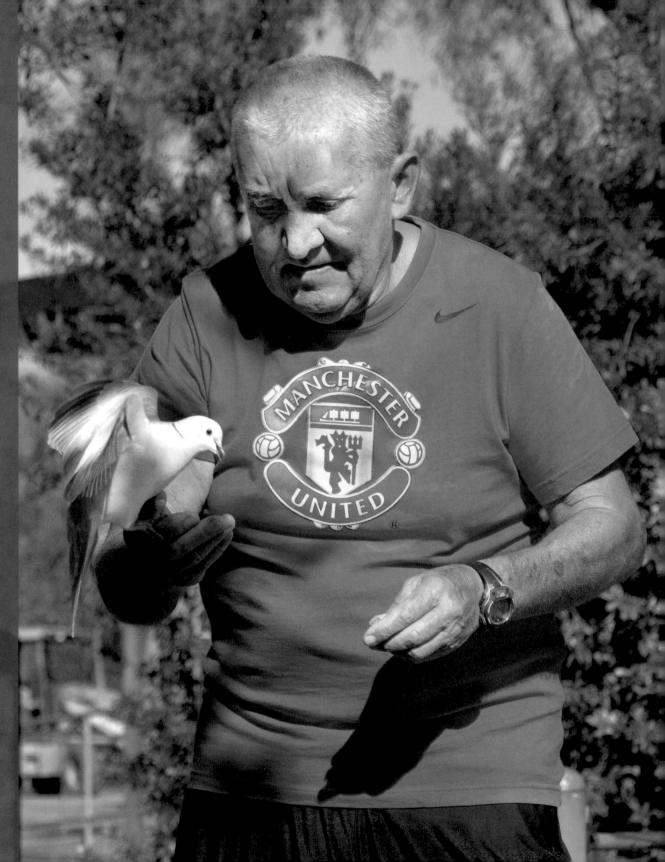

Some people call me Saint Francis because I am friends with the animals. I wonder if my being born in a barn was a precursor to my relationship with the critters at the Park.

BOB BUNOZA

I was born in Croatia in 1944, just before the end of World War II. A cannon hit the side of our house while my mom was in labor, and snow started pouring into the bedroom. My dad had to carry my mom to a barn, where I was born a couple hours later. Some people at Memorial Park call me Saint Francis because I am friends with the animals. I wonder if my being born in a barn was a precursor to my relationship with the critters at the Park.

In the 1960s, Croatia was controlled by Yugoslavia and anti-American sentiment was on the rise. I supported Croat independence and longed to escape the harsh socialist controls and relocate to the United States. I moved to New York City, but disappointment quickly set in. In Croatia I had seen a show on television of an American father coming downstairs in the morning to his family, who were waiting in a large living room. However, in New York, I had a tiny apartment and had to spend an hour every night fighting for a parking spot.

After eight years in New York, I decided to move to Houston because a friend promised I could get a job there. To my delight, I found a large, furnished apartment that overlooked a swimming pool and had my very own assigned, covered parking spot for the same price I had paid for my tiny New York apartment. I felt like I was the wealthiest man in the world.

When I moved to Houston, I played soccer and ran at Memorial Park on a regular basis. The *Houston Chronicle* posted race results every Thursday, and I started seeing names I recognized. I knew I could beat the men who were listed in the newspaper, so I decided to enter a 5K.

I competed in races throughout Houston for about ten years and usually finished in the second group of runners, not the winners, but the group that was just after the leaders. There were many days at the Park when I would do my tempo runs with the faster runners who were out for their easy runs.

I finished the 1992 Houston Marathon in three hours, twenty-six minutes. I wanted to race in another marathon so I could break the three-hour mark, but I kept getting hurt. I should have been satisfied to run just one marathon. Years passed before I finally went to the doctor. He told me I needed to give up running and just walk. It broke my heart to hear his diagnosis, but I knew he was right.

Over the years, I feel like I have developed a knack for recognizing individuals at the Park who have the potential to run much faster. I have helped many girls and one man achieve their best times after they agreed to follow my program. The most important rule is *no stopping*. Many people walk when they get tired, but if I can convince them to push through the initial desire to walk and catch their breath, then they can see drastic improvements.

Another part of my program includes running around the Park in a clockwise direction. By running clockwise, there is a long, gradual downhill on Memorial Drive and then a short, steep uphill. This is better for maintaining momentum compared to running in the opposite direction and being slowed down by a lengthy ascent.

I have been feeding the birds and squirrels at the Park for the last ten years. My friend was doing the same thing at his house and told me I should try it at the Park. However, I was hesitant because I was afraid I would eat the peanuts myself and gain weight. The first time I fed them, I was surprised at how friendly the animals were and how they seemed to trust me.

Now, when I get to the Park, I sit at the triangle-shaped median across the street from the driving range. I have named this spot Cro-Tex, which is short for Croatia-Texas. I give my birds and squirrels roasted, unsalted peanuts because the salted ones dirty my hands. I call all of the squirrels "Dog." There is a large white pigeon I named "White Boy" and a black-and-white one I call "Oreo."

The pigeons and doves are friendly. They don't hesitate to perch on my hand or stand in my lap. The black grackles have slowly warmed up to me, and there is even one that will stand on my head and wait for me to feed it. The squirrels come very close to me but do not usually eat directly out of my hand.

When I sit down at Cro-Tex, there are a couple of pigeons that peck my arm, hit me with their wing, and make a soft, throaty cooing sound if I do not feed them in a timely manner. They are just like spoiled children. I usually leave the Park with blood on my arms where the pigeons have poked me with their beaks.

People at the Park have many different names for me: St. Francis, Mr. Park, Bird Man, and Mayor of Memorial Park are a few I have heard. I sponsored a brick in front of the Tennis Center that says, "Bob Bunoza, Croatian Sensation, Mr. Park."

Once I had the privilege of running at the Park with President George H.W. Bush. As we were making our way around the trail, many people said, "Hello!" to me. After this happened several times, another runner told the President, "You are the President of the United States, but did you know you are running with the Mayor of Memorial Park?"

"Life is for participating, not for spectating."

KATHRINE SWITZER

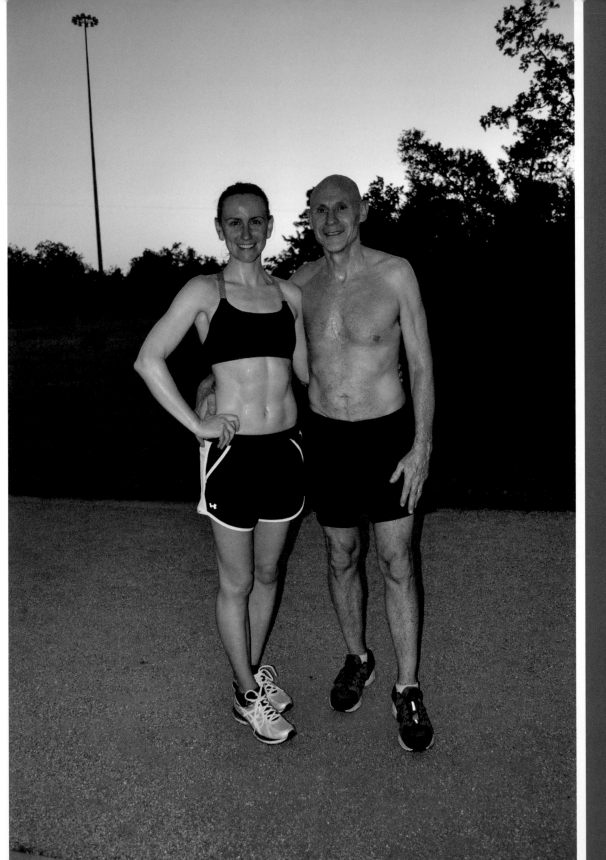

The morning of the marathon, I walked up to the starting line, found Wayne, and introduced myself. To my surprise, he lay on the ground, stuck his foot up in the air, and asked me to stretch his hammy.

WAYNE AND OLYA COHEN

Wayne and I grew up on opposite sides of the globe and had very different experiences that led us to Houston. Wayne was born in South Africa as tensions were rising and citizens were seeking every opportunity to flee the country. Believing there was no future for himself or his family, he sold his business and left the volatile, apartheid-ridden nation.

I grew up in Russia during the collapse of the Soviet Union, but my childhood memories eschew politics. What I do remember is how my dad occasionally took me on a six-mile jog near our house. At the end of each run, he would exclaim, "Wasn't that great?" While I loved spending time with my father, continuous running left me exhausted and nauseated. I could not identify with his love of the sport, but I dutifully faked my enthusiasm.

Wayne grew up playing cricket, soccer, and rugby and was accustomed to running to stay in shape. Shortly after he turned forty, a lifelong friend from South Africa was tragically killed in a car accident. Wayne was devastated and decided to run a marathon as a tribute to his friend. The following year, another lifelong friend died while riding his bike, and Wayne trained for another marathon. A year later, Wayne completed his third marathon to commemorate his dad's passing. Thankfully, Wayne has not had to endure another tragic loss, but twenty years and forty-five marathons later, he is still racing.

While Wayne was completing his third marathon, I moved from Russia to Tennessee and enrolled in college. I found myself overwhelmed by all of the new experiences: the language, culture, food, and even general attitude of Americans were very different from my home. I started running because it felt familiar and gave me something I could control. At the time, I ran at 4:00 a.m., thinking I was too slow to run in public.

Although I had never entered a race, I had a brilliant idea to enter a marathon. A training schedule I found on the Internet included track workouts and tempo runs. I had no idea what those were and opted to simply follow the suggested mileage. On race day, I expected to finish dead last but ended up being the third overall woman. However, as soon as I crossed the finish line, I had to drive to the emergency room because I had stress fractures in both of my legs. Despite the exhaustion and pain, my father's voice echoed in my mind and I thought, *That was great!* I could not wait to do it again.

When Wayne was training for his first marathon, he went to a local running store and asked about finding a group that he could run with. The director of the Houston Marathon was also in the store and suggested Wayne join Houston Fit, which met at Memorial Park every Saturday morning.

Wayne became close friends with many other athletes from that group, and they decided to continue running on their own a few years later. They called the group Wayne's Wankers and met at the Park several times each week. As the unofficial club grew, Wayne started sending out a newsletter with bits of information about anything he thought was relevant or funny. The distribution grew to 140 people, and there was a core group of about forty who trained together every week. One of his favorite lines, which he included in most newsletters, was a reminder for current group members to "Recruit the babes!"

A couple years after my first marathon, I moved to California and enrolled in graduate school. An Olympic Trials competitor invited me to run with her. She gave me confidence and assured me I was fast enough to train in the daylight. Upon completion of my degree, I obtained a job in Houston as an interpreter for NASA.

I moved in the middle of the summer and quickly realized that running in the Houston heat required careful planning and several water fountains. Although I lived and worked in the Clear Lake area, a coworker suggested that running on a soft, shaded trail in Memorial Park might be a good option. It did not take long before driving an hour to the Park became a part of my daily routine. I loved the atmosphere, and it motivated me to train harder.

Even before we officially met, Wayne saw me running at the Park and began calling me the "Russian Spy." Meanwhile, I heard about him from other runners; it seemed that everyone knew him. I was preparing for the upcoming Houston Marathon and being coached by Sean Wade, who leads the Kenyan Way training group. Sean pointed Wayne out and suggested I run the marathon with him because we were both shooting for similar finishing times, and Wayne was skilled at maintaining a steady pace.

The morning of the marathon, I found Wayne and introduced myself. To my surprise, he lay on the ground, stuck his foot up in the air, and asked me to stretch his hammy. Despite that abrupt beginning, Wayne was a gentleman during the race and made sure to always grab enough water for both of us. I finished a minute ahead of Wayne, and when we reunited after the race, he insisted I join the Wankers.

A few weeks later, at one of the Wankers' weekday runs, Wayne pulled me aside after the workout. It was March 8, which is known as International Women's Day in Russia. Wayne told me he had a gift, and I was shocked he even knew about the holiday. However, I became very confused when I opened the beautifully wrapped package to find a single loaf of bread. It turned out that Wayne had been researching the holiday. Apparently, it commemorates an event during the destitute times of World War I when Russian women went on strike for "Bread and Peace." I was slightly embarrassed because I had just been schooled in my birth country's history. But I was also very impressed.

Wayne continued to impress me with his unwavering dedication to the sport as well as his kind heart. He was the first member of the group to break three hours in a marathon, and everyone was extremely proud of him. Although my interest in him grew, Wayne had not yet passed my test. One of the last things my family told me before I moved to the United States was to never get serious with a guy who does not attend the ballet or opera. With that in mind, I invited Wayne to the opera, and to my delight, he agreed. A few years later, we were married.

We still both love running and want to be able to continue well into our eighties. After many injuries, it became clear that if we kept pushing ourselves to run a personal best every year, our running days would be numbered. It took some time, but our goals were readjusted. Today, we run because we enjoy being outdoors, staying active, and catching up with our friends at Memorial Park.

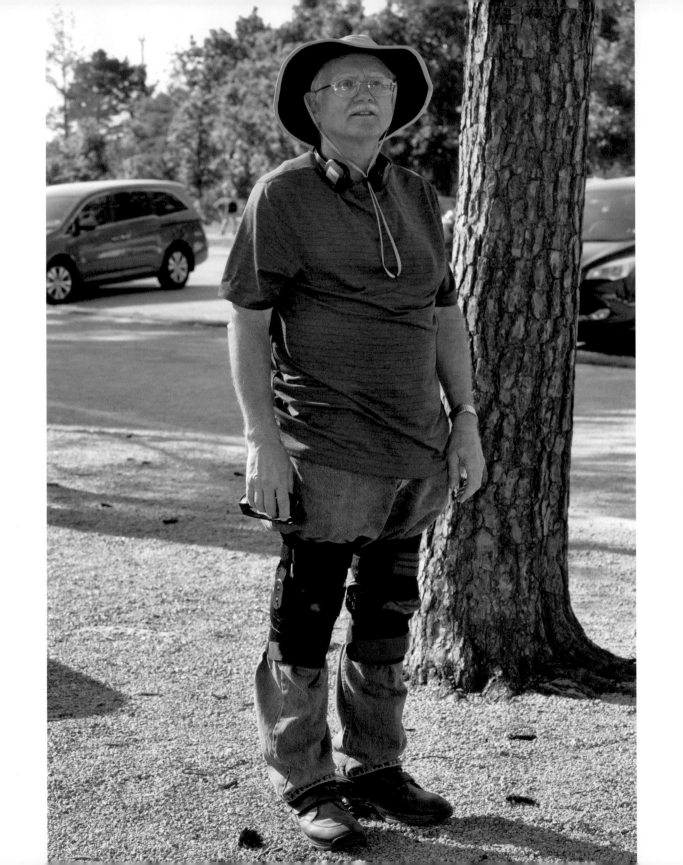

CHARLES CUPP

I try to walk at Memorial Park for two hours each day. My wife has cancer, and I feel like I should be diligent about donating blood, as she has relied on donors to stay alive. However, I struggle to keep my red blood cell count up high enough to be able to give blood on a regular basis. My doctor told me that drinking beet juice would help to raise my hemoglobin, but I hate the way it tastes. I finally figured out that if I mix half a bottle of Diet Dr. Pepper with the beet juice, it does not taste so bad. When I am at the Park, I always carry my Diet Dr. Pepper/beet juice concoction with me when I walk. After I finally get it down, I just refill the bottle with water so I can stay hydrated.

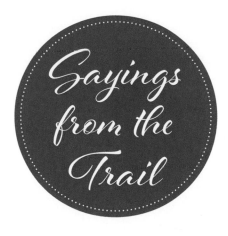

"Do you want to meet at the zero, stretching deck, gazebo, pool, or Running Trails Center?"

There are many places to meet at the Park. The zero-mile marker in front of the Tennis Center is the most popular spot, but these other locations also have easy access to water fountains, restrooms, and parking.

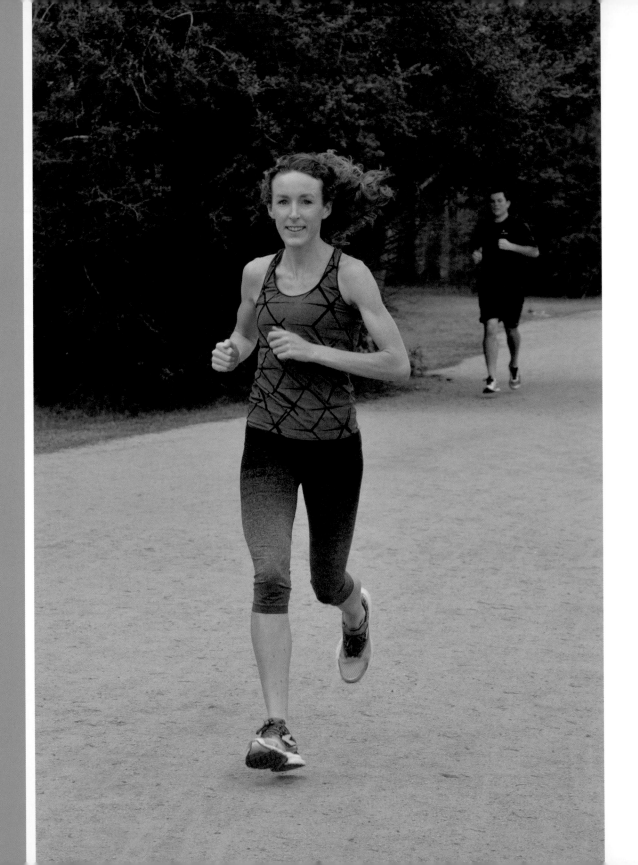

When I was training for the World Championships Marathon, I placed my water bottles on a table in the grass and put a box about a hundred meters away. I also posted signs that said, "Marathon training in progress. Please do not touch."

MARY DAVIES

I grew up in a tiny town in New Zealand and have fond memories of playing at the white, sandy beach that was two minutes away from my home. After high school, I played field hockey but also enjoyed running on my own, when I had time. My field hockey coach finally contacted a local running coach and asked for his help. She told him that she had an athlete who liked to run, but unfortunately she did not know what to do with me. I was happy for her to reach out because I did not have a clue what I was doing.

Within a year, I was winning local races and was excited to see such dramatic improvements in my times. A girl from New Zealand who was running at Oklahoma State University heard about my success and suggested the coach there contact me. After a brief phone call, he flew to New Zealand and visited our home. It was surreal to have him sitting in our living room, speaking with my family about racing in the United States. Until that point, I had barely left the country. It all happened so fast, but the next thing I knew, I was on a plane headed to Oklahoma.

When I left New Zealand, we all assumed I would spend four years in Oklahoma and then come back home. It sounded like an exciting adventure, but then I met my husband. He is originally from Brazil and was studying for his PhD. We both never dreamed of living in the United States after graduation, but his plan was to become a doctor and move back to Brazil, not New Zealand. I would still like to live there again someday. The lifestyle is more relaxed, and my family is there. For now though, my husband has a wonderful job in Houston, and we are fortunate to be able to travel home frequently.

We moved to Houston in 2008, and I was shocked when the summer heat made me feel like I was running in a sauna. My husband initially brought me to Memorial Park because he had played tennis there and knew I would enjoy running on the trail. I thought the trees made the Park a beautiful place to run and liked that I did not have to worry about stoplights.

Since I first ran at the Park eight years ago, I have met so many friendly people. I worked out around the same time each day and started recognizing other regulars. I felt like I got to know them, but the funny thing is, I never actually spoke to them. I was also introduced to a few of the local elite runners who trained at the Park. It was nice to have a group of athletes who were training at the same pace as me.

By 2009, I was trying to qualify for the World Championships Marathon in Berlin. I preferred to do my twenty-mile long runs at the Park even though the loops were repetitive. The Park allowed me to concentrate on completing each mile at an exact speed while focusing on maintaining my form. It was perfect for that intense training because I did not have to worry about dodging traffic and could approach the workouts as if they were races.

I also tried to simulate the refreshment stops that would be at the upcoming World Championships. I placed my water bottles on a table in the grass adjacent to the trail. Then I put a box about a hundred meters away from the table where I could drop the empty bottles. I also posted signs that said, "Marathon training in progress. Please do not touch." As I zoomed around the Park at six minutes per mile for twenty miles, it was funny how many comments I received. People would see me grabbing the bottles and ask what I was doing. After I explained the reasoning behind the table and box, they seemed excited about my upcoming race and encouraged me.

I finished thirty-fourth at the World Championships in a time of two hours, thirty-eight minutes, and forty-eight seconds. That time was four minutes slower than my personal best, but it was also eighty-five degrees at the start. For the first time, I found myself thankful for being able to train in Houston. Most of the other runners were complaining about how hot it was, but I remained calm and felt like I had an advantage, having figured out how to survive Houston's heat.

I had my son in 2011 and my daughter in 2014. When I was pregnant, I jogged to stay fit but did not do any intense training. My mother-in-law still lives in Brazil, but her only grandchildren are here in Houston, so she comes to visit us quite often. It is always nice to have her help because I get the chance to train more intensely for the few weeks she is visiting. I do not run with my kids in a stroller because I think it would be difficult to concentrate. Also, any time we are out, they would rather walk than sit in a stroller.

After my son was born, I would come to the Park every other day while he was at daycare. Now that I also have my daughter, it has not been as easy for me to squeeze in the extra time it takes to drive to and from the Park. Occasionally I am able to make it there, but for the most part I usually just run near my house. I do miss the people and atmosphere of the Park, but I have also found that having children has given me a totally different perspective on running.

Before I was a mom, my attitude toward training and racing was unhealthy. Running consumed me, and my entire focus was on how well I performed. My attitude was determined by how the workout had gone that day, and my poor husband had to endure constant mood swings. It was terrible. I was close to quitting running because it was not even fun, but thankfully my husband encouraged me to keep going. He suggested that I could try to not be so stressed out about it, which seemed almost unfathomable at the time. But then, a couple months later, I became pregnant.

After I had my son, I decided to try running again but as a hobby. To my surprise, I found myself racing really well. I do not know if I became physically stronger after becoming a mom, but I definitely feel like I became mentally stronger. I realized there are other things in life that are more important. My children are my main focus now, and I schedule my workouts around them. I know running is not the main thing. It is still important to me, but I have found a balance.

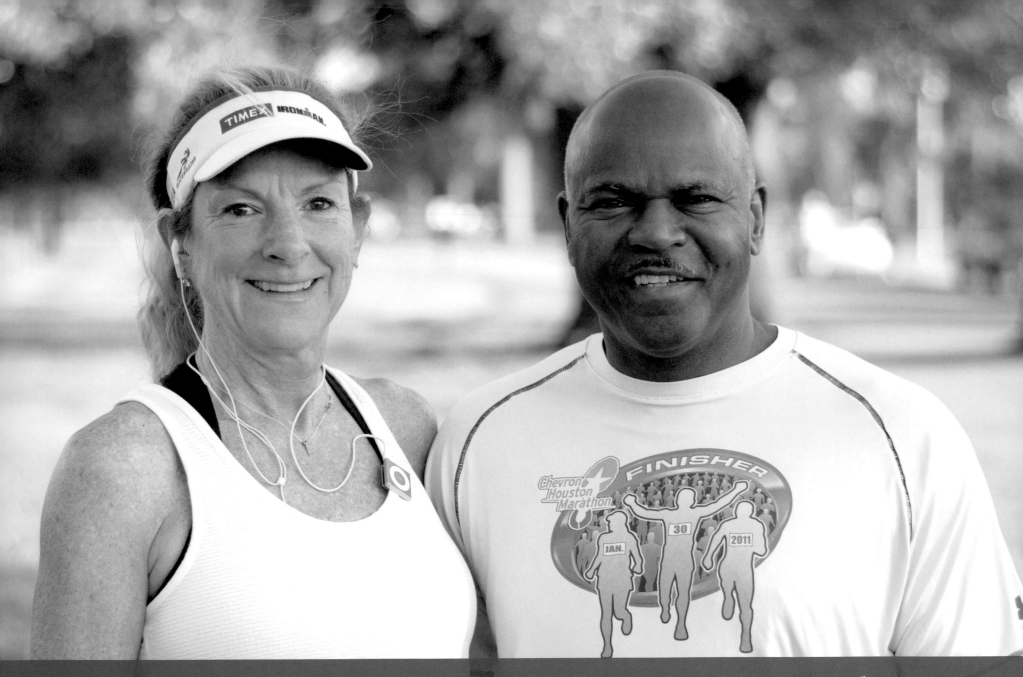

One morning in 2001, I met my "running boyfriend," Larry Mosley.
We have spent countless hours training together while discussing our personal
lives, running, work, or anything else we were going through.

MERRY DAVIS

My running career began in 1994, a few years after I sobered up. I had never been athletic until that time in my life, but I needed to find something to replace all the damaging things I had been doing with my spare time. I lived about a mile away from Memorial Park and decided to venture out to the trail and try running. In the beginning, even though I was only doing a few miles each day, I was surprised and excited to see my body changing as I lost weight. Also, I was thrilled to be able to finish a 5K, which was unimaginable a few years earlier. I was hooked, and running quickly became the "other addiction."

When I started, I always wore coordinating outfits. My jog bras and running shorts had vibrant patterns that were perfectly matched. Not only were they color coordinated; they also had to be the same brand. I would have never been seen in a Nike shirt and Asics shorts, regardless of the colors. Now that I look back on that attitude, I think it was really silly. Who cares? I guess I did at the time.

My life has been enriched by my running at Memorial Park in ways that I cannot begin to enumerate. The Park is simply the best thing that ever happened to me. Although I had given up drinking a few years before I started running, I was still struggling to quit smoking. Every day after work, I would run a loop at the Park and then sit on the tailgate of my Ford Explorer to smoke a cigarette. It never crossed my mind that the smoke might be an imposition upon the other runners who walked by my truck. In 1996, I was finally able to quit smoking, and the next thing I knew I was running the River Oaks ten-mile loop every weekend. The joy of being able to complete such long distances gave me great pride, and I began to wonder what I ever did before I became a runner.

In 2000, I was one of the founding members of the Memorial Park Running Club (MPRC). I ran at the Park at least three days a week, early in the morning, and did my long runs with the other members of the club on Saturday mornings. The MPRC lasted for about eight years, and by then a handful of members had served as president at least two times each. The new members who were coming in were not as interested in contributing the time and energy that was necessary to keep the club going, so we disbanded around 2008 and applied the remaining money toward a brick that was laid near the entrance of the Tennis Center.

One morning in 2001, as I was getting ready to start my regular 5:00 a.m. easy run, I met Larry Mosley. Although he lived and worked in southeast Houston, he had been making the thirty-minute drive to and from the Park every morning since 1976. We quickly hit it off, and for the last fifteen years, I have referred to Larry as my "running boyfriend." We have spent countless hours training together while discussing our personal lives, running, work, or anything else we were going through.

There were many days when I was busy helping the MPRC, and I would not get my usual chance to spend time running with and talking to Larry. I would find myself longing to get back to the Park the following day so we could catch up on whatever we had missed during the previous run. He is the best friend I have ever had in the running community. We still talk about being able to run when we are old, no matter what it takes.

After running for twenty years, I have accumulated a laundry list of injuries: two stress fractures, two knee surgeries, three cervical disk fusions, lumbar surgery, rotator cuff surgery, plantar fasciitis, black toenails, and calloused feet. Yet running is still the medicine that soothes my soul. I have graduated to Hoka shoes now so that I can continue this madness with as little impact as possible.

I recently moved to Katy, which is about twenty miles from the Park. There are an abundance of gyms, school tracks, and exercise paths at several nearby parks. However, nothing compares to the experiences I had at Memorial Park when I was a regular there. I still get over to the Park to run with Larry from time to time, and it becomes even more obvious to me the gem of a place that it is. I miss it terribly, along with all the familiarity it holds.

I am glad it is there not only for me but also for the entire city of Houston. I will always treasure the fond memories of the people and of the Park itself. I have never lost my gratitude for what a beautiful place we have to run, socialize, and burn off stress. I still believe the Memorial Park and Buffalo Bayou areas are some of the most beautiful things Houston has to offer.

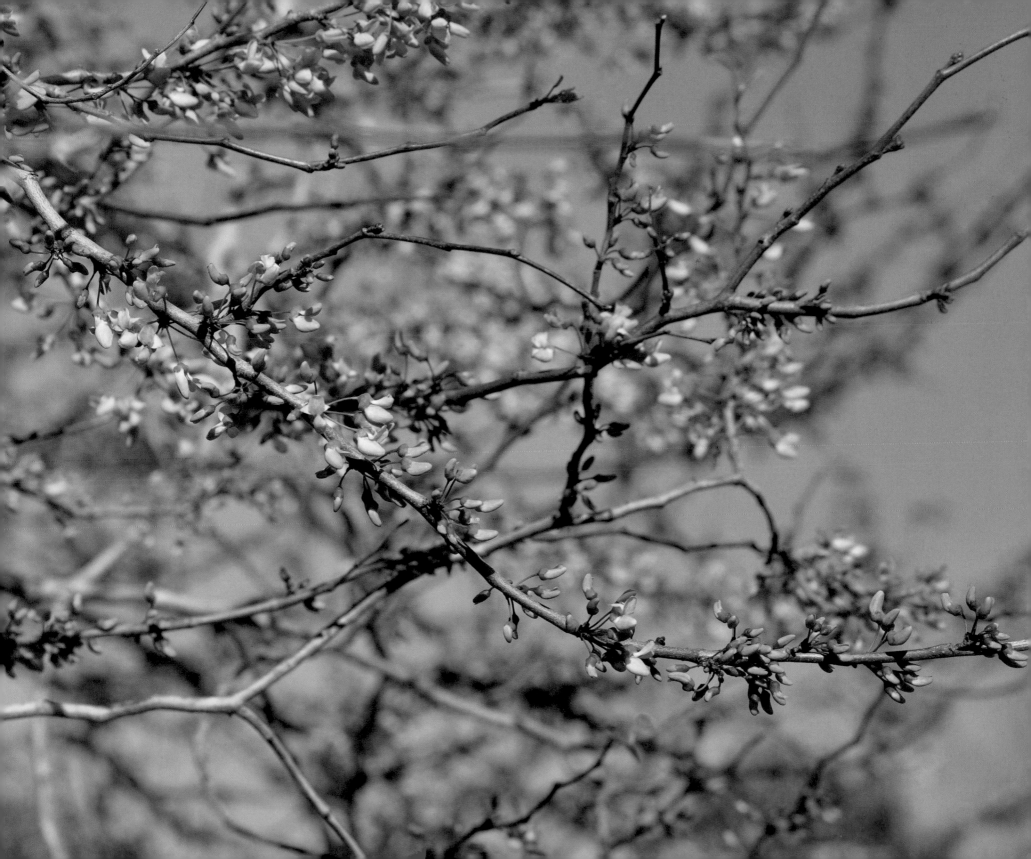

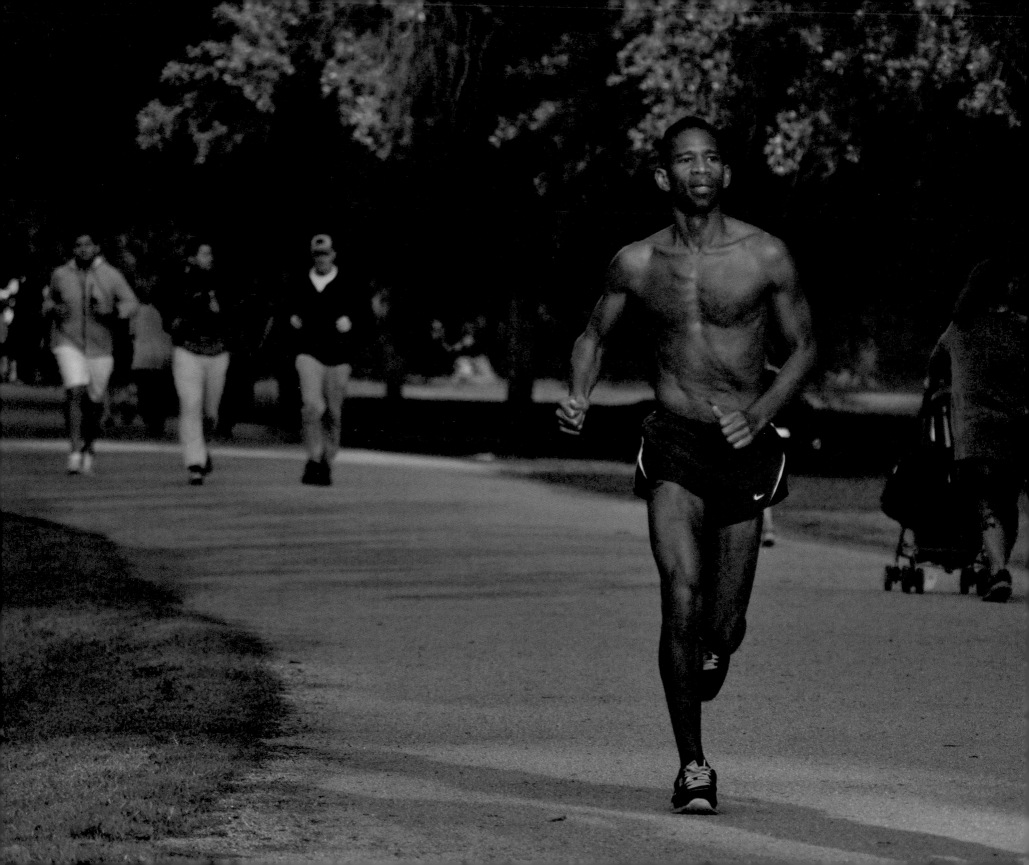

CARLO DEASON

started running in Memorial Park in the late 1990s. My training shoe of choice has always been the Reebok Classic because of its ability to take a high level of impact during my long-distance training runs. I have tried other brands, but Reebok is the best shoe for me. For my actual races, I switch to the lightest-weight Nike running flats I can find.

I enjoy competing in local, state, national, and international road races, cross-country meets, and track meets. My goal is to place in the top three in my age group (forty-five to forty-nine years old) at every race. I feel extremely fortunate that the vast majority of my vacations have been to international locations including Australia, Europe, Central America, and Canada. With each trip, I like to compete in road races or track meets one week and then sightsee the following week.

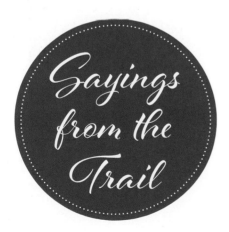

"You go clockwise, and I will go counterclockwise until I meet you."
"Wait! Which direction is clockwise?"

When someone in the group is late, the others will usually start running in one direction and then have the latecomer run in the opposite direction until they meet. This type of discussion usually ends with, "When I stand on the trail and look at the Tennis Center, do I go to the right or left?"

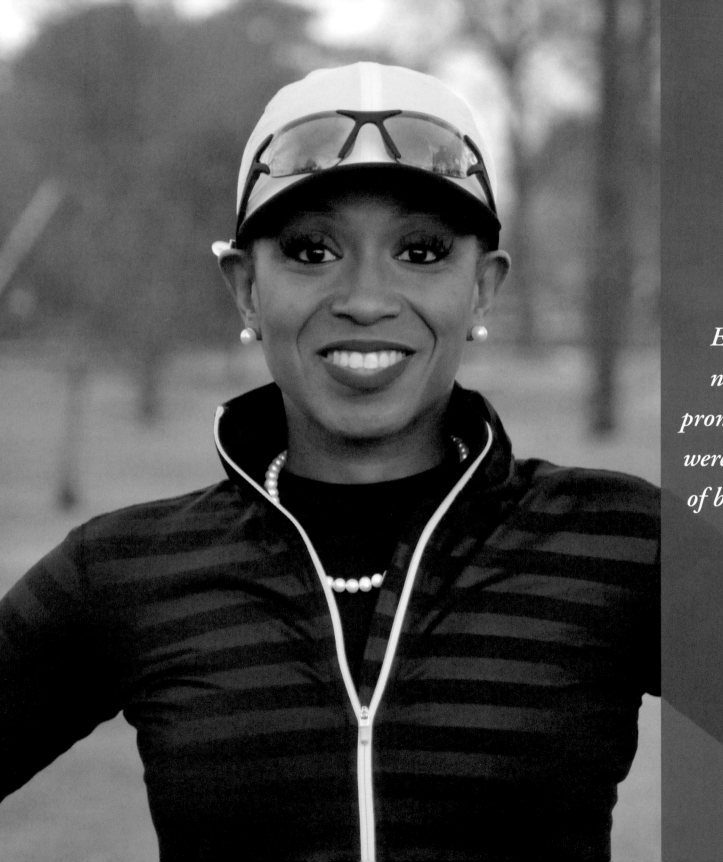

Even though I had never run before, I promised myself that if I were ever able to get out of bed, I would finish a marathon.

CRYSTAL HADNOTT

Many people know me as the girl whose destiny was shaped by an accident, but as I reflect on the last ten years of my life, I know it was much more than an accident that led me to where I am today. Shortly after I graduated from college, I was walking through my office at work when I suddenly slipped and fell. The injury caused severe nerve damage, which led to paralysis in my hip and leg. I was forced to lie in bed for six weeks, and my muscles began to atrophy. I relied on my friends and family to carry me anywhere I needed to go.

Even though I had never run before, I promised myself that if I were ever able to get out of bed, I would finish a marathon. I had no idea what that meant or what would be required, but I was desperate to be able to move again.

I slowly regained feeling in my leg and was sent to a physical therapist to learn how to walk again. After working for a month, I progressed to walking with a cane, but each step was a constant battle to maintain balance. Just a few weeks after I had secretly promised myself I would complete a marathon, I was stunned when the therapist warned me I would never be able to run. He cautioned me that I had achieved as much as I could ever hope. At the time, I was twenty-six years old and my first thought was, *Walking with a cane is not sexy!*

Even though I do not recommend this, I walked out of his office and never went back. I began reading books about the body and healing. I also visited several physical-therapy offices throughout Houston to see what type of equipment they used. Many of them had Pilates reformer machines, so I researched how to use the machine and started working out on my own. After two months, I was excited to feel my body change as I became stronger.

I decided to set a goal for myself so I would have something to work toward. I was still walking with a cane and fell every time I tried to run. Despite my slow progress, I entered the Marine Corps Marathon, which was nine months away. When I began learning how to run, I would go to the trail at Hermann Park. There was an older gentleman, Mr. Marvin Taylor, who knew what I was working toward. Each time he saw me fall, he would encourage me to get back up and try again. When I was finally able to complete two miles without falling, I decided I was ready to run at Memorial Park.

I was terrified the first time I drove to Memorial Park because I had the perception it was a place where only fast runners trained. However, I quickly realized there was a tremendous community of athletes who were willing to help me even though I was new to the sport. My longest run before the Marine Corps Marathon was thirteen miles, but the thrill of finishing left me yearning to continue. I also decided that I needed to move closer to the Park so I could run there all the time.

Throughout my training I continued to do Pilates because it allowed me to maintain strength and improve my form. Eventually I became a certified instructor because I wanted to avoid paying for the classes. I enjoyed my full-time job as a lobbyist and never dreamed about doing anything else with the certification until my mom suddenly passed away in 2012. She was young and beautiful, and I looked up to her as my hero. She was my greatest cheerleader. I was in shock and decided to take a month off of work to process my heartache.

During that month off, I felt a strong urge to begin a career teaching Pilates. Just as I experienced when I signed up for my first marathon, I did not have any idea what would be required to earn a living as a trainer. However, I felt certain it was time for a change. I returned to work and informed my boss that I was resigning so I could teach Pilates. My coworkers wondered if I had lost my mind due to the stress of my mom's passing.

That Tuesday afternoon, as I walked out of my former employer's office, I posted an update on Facebook announcing that I was accepting clients for Pilates lessons. By the end of the day, I had five people who had scheduled appointments, and by the end of the week, I had met with ten more.

That weekend, I also received a call from KHOU Channel 11. One of my clients knew someone at the station who was looking for an expert on health and wellness. The client suggested they call me. Less than a week after I quit my job as a lobbyist, I was being interviewed on television as a nutrition and fitness specialist!

People often question why the name of my business (Synergy Total Holistic Health and Wellness) is so long. As I was standing there being interviewed, the newsman asked me for the name and website of my company. I had to make up something on the spot and knew it needed to be long enough that it would be impossible for the website address to have already been taken. As soon as we finished the interview, I rushed home to create a website before it aired that evening.

Today, I am Channel 11's expert on health and wellness, and my business is thriving. I enjoy working with runners who are looking to improve their stride and strength through Pilates. Over the last few years, a large portion of my work has been with individuals who have injuries, nerve damage, or orthopedic issues. Ironically, the same therapist who told me I would never walk without a cane now refers his clients to me.

Since that first race in 2006, I have completed fourteen full marathons and eighty half marathons. Every time I run, I wear bright red lipstick, pearl earrings, and a pearl necklace. I want to pay tribute to my mom, who was always dressed impeccably no matter what she was doing. I also like to say, "I run for those who can't." I feel like I can honor my mom and my clients who are in the same situation I was ten years ago. I know what it feels like to yearn to run even though someone says it is impossible.

People have forgotten how to tell a story. Stories don't have a middle or an end anymore. They usually have a beginning that never stops beginning.

STEVEN SPIELBERG

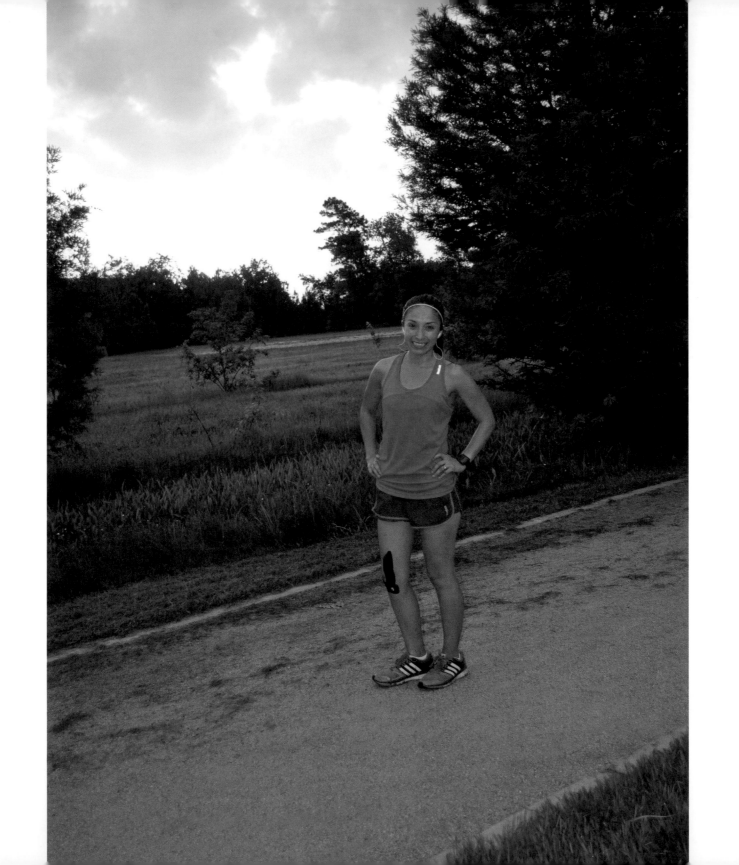

ELVIRA HALL

I live in Katy but make the forty-five-minute drive to Memorial Park because my coach, Al Lawrence, is there. Also, the Park is a great place for me to find other fast women to run with. I am a teacher and like to get my workouts in before school, which means I have to start running at 4:00 a.m. At first I was nervous about coming to the Park that early, but I quickly met another girl who was always there at the same time. I asked if she was scared to be at the Park by herself. She replied, "No, because I am not alone. I run with God!" We hit it off and run together regularly. As we make our way around the trail, we pray for the people we see and ask God to bless them.

"They say you become who you hang out with. Well I can tell you for sure, you made me a better man."

TOBY MAC

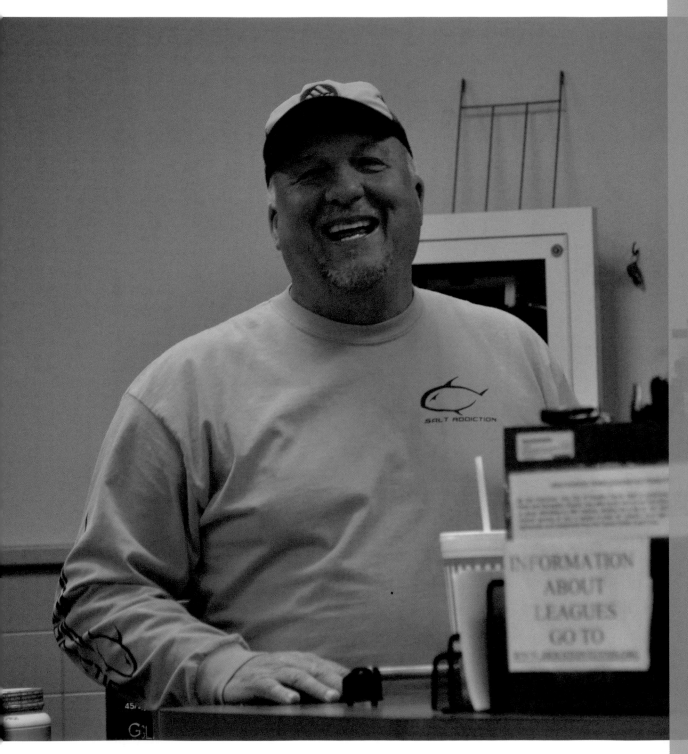

I received a call from someone who asked to schedule a tennis lesson. I almost lost my breath when I finally realized he was the same guy I had seen on the news because he was on trial for murder!

OTIS JOHNSON

I started working at the Memorial Park Tennis Center in 1980. We were working out of a temporary trailer because the previous tennis center had burned down in 1977, and it took several years for the new building to be completed. The parking lot was lined with Porta-Potties since the restrooms were not available, but many people also used the Porta-Potties as dressing rooms to change into their exercise clothes after work. I found great humor in watching a few plump individuals cram themselves and their duffle bags into the narrow stalls. I can only imagine the contortions they put their oversized bodies through in those tiny compartments. There is no doubt they were warmed up and ready to exercise when they finally emerged.

Another interesting memory from the early 1980s involved a man who raced around the Park barefoot. People started complaining because he also smoked a cigarette while running. I guess he was trying to finish the loop before his cigarette was out, or maybe he decided that because he couldn't give up smoking, he would incorporate running to counteract the damages of tobacco. I'm still not sure how the absence of shoes played into his plans. Unfortunately, I could not do anything about the complaints, as it was legal to smoke in city parks at that time.

There was a day in the late 1990s when a man came in the Tennis Center and asked for tape. He said he had some photos he wanted to assemble so he could make a collage. I thought his request was strange but knew we had a roll of tape in the storage room. As I was rummaging through the closet, a lady in the Smoothie King line began screaming. Apparently the man had covered the table next to our cash register with the photographs he wanted to tape together, and she was horrified when she saw that they were all pornographic pictures of women. I cannot remember if I ever found the tape, because the next thing I knew, he was shoving the photos back in his envelope and sprinting out the door.

When I became the tennis pro in 1997, I kept track of my clients' workouts and schedules in a spiral-bound notebook. Today I use a computer, but regardless of whom I am meeting, I still love helping people improve their skills. I have coached a wide range of individuals, from those who are picking up a racket for the first time to world-class players who have retired but want to get back into shape.

I was shocked the first time I worked with a former professional player. There is an astounding difference between a typical client and a professional. When he hit the ball, it was like a rocket had been launched off his racket. Playing with him gave me a new perspective on the game of tennis. Not only were his movements quicker and his strength greater, but even his vision was better. He could react to any ball I hit as soon as it left my racket. I think that difference can also be seen on the trail at the Park. There are athletes who can maintain a five-minute, thirty-second-per-mile pace for an entire marathon, and there are people who struggle to walk one mile in less than thirty minutes.

A few years after I became the tennis pro, I received an intriguing call from someone who asked to schedule a lesson. I kept thinking his name sounded familiar, so I finally looked him up. I almost lost my breath when I realized he was the same guy I had seen on the news because he was on trial for murder! I worked to be professional and behave the same way I do around all of my clients. I guess he was satisfied with his lesson because he scheduled another one a couple days later. Shortly after the second lesson, he was acquitted of murder, and I never heard from him again. He tipped me $10 each time, which made me thankful I was still on his good side.

After working at the Tennis Center for many years, one thing I have learned is to set a folded towel on the counter where customers can place their money. Some may think the towel is there to absorb the moisture from sweaty runners. The actual reason is because a few individuals insist on slamming their money on the counter, even though I have pleaded with them to stop. I dreaded seeing those customers walk up because that meant I would soon be chasing coins as they bounced across the floor. I finally realized if I place a towel on the counter, it keeps the coins from rolling off the desk when the money is slammed down.

In addition to working at the Tennis Center, I have also enjoyed jogging around the Park for the last thirty-five years. My favorite memory of working out on the trail is from 1980, when a frigid storm blew through Houston and we had two inches of snow on the ground. The temperature had dropped into the single digits, and my friend and I were bundled up like we were on the North Pole. The Park was covered with fresh, untouched snow, and every step we took left a perfect footprint that looked like something you would see on a Christmas card.

As we made our way around the trail in this serene, peaceful setting, we were not surprised to eventually see another runner coming toward us along Memorial Drive. We soon realized that, in typical Memorial Park fashion, he was only wearing tennis shoes and running shorts. We had a good laugh as we continued along the trail. The people who exercise at the Park never seem to change. They are all unique in their own ways!

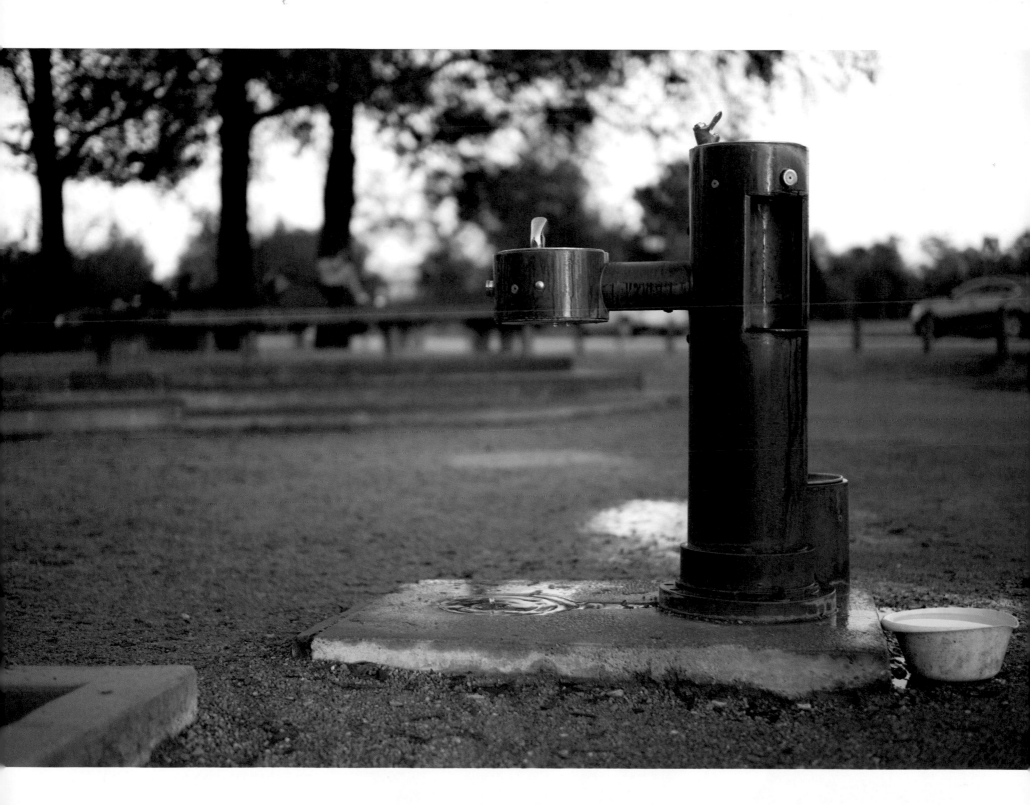

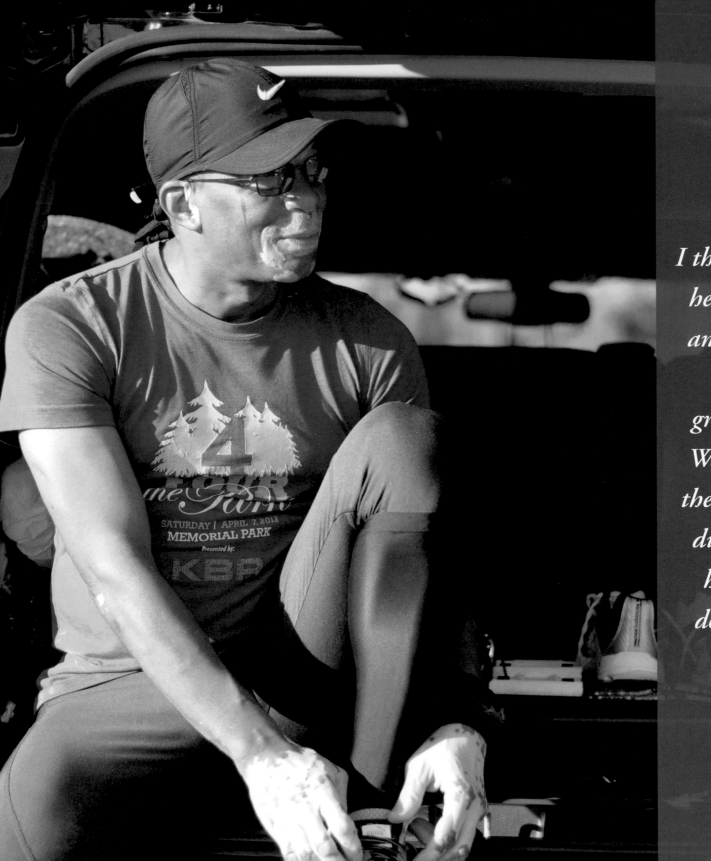

I think most people have heard of Camp Logan and how the Park was used as a training ground during World War I. Unfortunately, there was another event during that time that has not been passed down as it should be.

RODNEY JOHNSON

I grew up in the First Ward, north of downtown Houston. At that time, there was poverty on every corner, and everyone I knew was struggling just to make ends meet. In junior high, a coach encouraged me to join the track team. Later that year, a volunteer at the Wesley Community Center took a few of us to run at Memorial Park. On the way home, he drove the bus through River Oaks, and I saw the possibilities life offers.

By the time we made it back to the First Ward that evening, I felt as if the Park was a million miles away from my home. Up to that point, the only place I had ever run was on a quarter-mile track, and I had definitely never seen a house that had more than three bedrooms. After I graduated from high school, a friend invited me to run with her at the Park. It was only then that I realized I could get on I-10 and be there in five minutes, as opposed to the million-miles-away memory I had from my youth.

I have been a regular at the Park for thirty years. Today, most people recognize me as the guy who sits on the back of his Jeep Cherokee. I always park at one of the spots that overlooks the trail to the left of the Tennis Center. Occasionally I have to wait for a space to open up, but I do not mind. Those few, select spots allow me to watch everyone who runs by and still see the stretching area. There is always something going on.

A few people call me the Mayor of the Park because I know or at least recognize almost everyone. I also pay attention to how they relate to each other. I think it is odd to see people running alone. To me, the Park is a social place where you go to be with other athletes. Some tell me they actually prefer to run by themselves, but to me that is just strange.

I always have several pairs of sparkling-clean running shoes lined up in the back of my truck. I choose which pair I want to wear depending on my workout. After each run, I clean the shoes so they look as if I have pulled them out of the box for the very first time. I also chew gum and wear headphones when I run, even though I do not usually listen to music. I have become accustomed to having them with me and feel like something is missing if I run without them.

I think most people have heard of Camp Logan and how the Park was used as a training ground during World War I. Unfortunately, there was another event during that time that has not been passed down as it should be. When Camp Logan was under construction, African American soldiers from Chicago were assigned to guard the site. The men had stellar military reputations and were accustomed to being treated with respect. However, the Jim Crow laws of the South were still in effect in Houston, and many citizens were upset that the men were given such authority and responsibility.

Rumors began circulating throughout the camp that a police officer had killed one of the soldiers. They also thought a group of armed Houstonians was heading their way to take out any other soldiers who tried to stand their ground. Overwhelmed with fear and panic, more than one hundred black soldiers left the campground and began marching through the streets of Houston. Sadly, twenty soldiers, citizens, and policemen were killed, and another nineteen soldiers were eventually executed after their military trial.

Although we talk about Camp Logan and World War I as if they were events that occurred in ancient history, my parents and grandparents grew up in the same hostile atmosphere that reigned during that time. They endured segregation and discrimination on a daily basis and always talked about how hard they worked to overcome their circumstances.

As I was growing up, I heard these stories and was proud of my strong heritage. I wanted to represent my family well and tried my best to please my parents. In 1989, I was home from college and went to my old high school to pick up my cousin. I did not know he had been arguing with some of his classmates who were also at the school. When I arrived, they started pushing me around. As I began to retaliate, I was stabbed several times. My friend rushed me to the fire station on Scott Street, where a paramedic kept screaming at me and insisting that I stay awake. He promised he would not let me die, but by the time the ambulance arrived at the hospital, I had lost a tremendous amount of blood and had a collapsed lung.

As I lay on the hospital bed and heard my mom crying, I was overwhelmed with sadness because I felt like I had disappointed my parents. I felt as though the strong heritage I had worked so hard to defend had been tarnished.

Even though I survived the night and am thankful to be alive, the scars on my back represent more than just a physical wound. Before I was stabbed, I was soft-spoken and had many friends. But that night, I changed. Today I am not afraid to express my opinion, because I feel I need to speak up for what is right.

Also, I realized that the reason I was attacked was because I was with my cousin. I learned to be extremely selective about who I associate with. Although most of the people at Memorial Park would say they know me, there are actually only a handful of them who I am really close to and hang out with away from the Tennis Center.

In the fall of 2015, my friends and I finished an eighteen-mile-long run on Saturday, but by the end of the following week, I felt so sick that I could not even run one mile. I went to the doctor and was shocked to find out that my pancreas had stopped producing insulin and my blood sugar was three times higher than the normal level. Even though I am thin, exercise regularly, eat healthier than anyone I know, and do not have a family history of diabetes, I was diagnosed with type 1 diabetes. Today, I wear an insulin pump and am working to figure out the best way to manage my disease while continuing to run long distances.

As I think about my brushes with death in 1989 and again in 2015, I have learned to appreciate each new day. I know I have a purpose and a responsibility to continue exercising, working hard, and living a life that would make my parents proud.

I love my job and find it rewarding to see my clients succeed. As a nutritionist, I enjoy working with endurance athletes because they are motivated to follow my recommendations, which makes it satisfying to see them succeed.

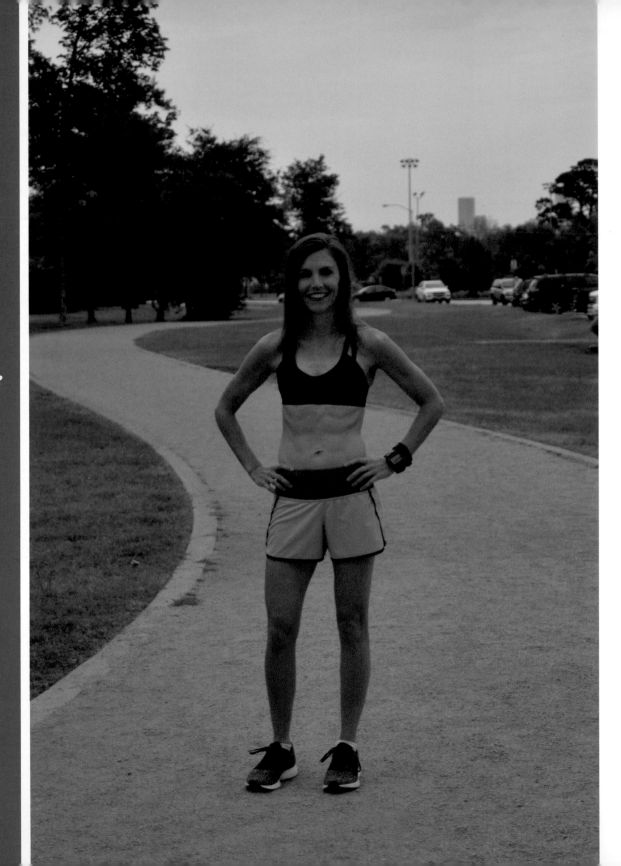

CATHERINE KRUPPA

I grew up in a very athletic family. My parents are both competitive tennis players and have completed many marathons. I was a gymnast through high school and then a diver at Texas A&M University, where I majored in nutrition. As a child, I occasionally ran with my parents but never more than a few miles. I got married in 1997 and moved to Houston. The company I worked for had a campaign to encourage employees to get in shape and hosted a time trial at Memorial Park. I thought it sounded like fun, but after they told us to start running, it did not take long for everyone to become spread out. I was nervous because I did not know where the path would lead and did not know anyone who was around me. I had no idea the Memorial Park trail was a loop.

By the end of the time trial, my fears were calmed, and I decided the Park would be a great place to exercise on a regular basis. As Memorial Park became a part of my daily routine, a running group began putting flyers on cars to advertise a training program for the 1999 Houston Marathon. I decided to join the group because I had watched my parents run in many marathons and knew I also wanted to finish one. I met three people in that group who I enjoyed running with, and we quickly became inseparable. In addition to the pride I felt after finishing my first marathon in four hours, twenty-seven minutes, I also treasure the wonderful memories of training with my friends. Although they have all moved away, we still get together on a regular basis. We recently met in Arizona to hike the Grand Canyon, and it was as if we had never been apart.

In 2011, I started my own business, Advice for Eating. I never viewed myself as an entrepreneur, and branching out on my own as a registered dietitian was very scary. To my delight, it has worked out very well, and the business is thriving. God has allowed me to grow more than I could have ever imagined. I love my job and find it very rewarding to see my clients succeed. As a registered dietitian, the majority of my clients come for advice on losing weight or finding a nutrition program to work with diseases, but my passion is working with endurance athletes. They are tremendously motivated to follow my recommendations, which makes it satisfying to see them succeed.

I try to encourage my weight-loss clients not to be intimidated if they decide to incorporate running into their routine. From my first marathon in 1999 to my fastest in 2011 when I finally broke the three-hour barrier, I dropped almost ninety minutes off my time. We all have to start somewhere. I advise people to set little goals and work to achieve them. It is more important to just start moving than to worry about trying to win the race.

I am also a big advocate of my clients getting outside, but that can be challenging in Houston. One of my clients recently began the Couch to 5K program, which encourages former couch potatoes to build up enough strength to finish a 5K. He was very new to walking and running and asked me to recommend a place for an exercise field trip. I suggested he try Memorial Park because I knew it would be very motivating to him, and there are people of every shape, size, and age. He asked where it was, which made my jaw drop. Memorial Park is my home away from home, and I was shocked to realize someone did not even know how to get there!

After running at the Park for almost nineteen years, I have definitely seen it change. I also think I have changed more than the Park has. After my three close friends moved away, I met another group of people who were all training for the St. George's Marathon. Suddenly, I went from being a social jogger to a serious runner. I was surprised that they did not talk during their tempo runs. It never dawned on me that I should occasionally run so hard that I could not talk. Of course, my times dropped dramatically after I began running with them.

In the beginning I worked out in the evenings, but after my son was born, I decided it was easier to fit running in my schedule if I started at five in the morning. This means I have to go to bed really, really early, but that is what it takes to be fit. I am a health professional and am constantly explaining how important sleep is to a person's overall wellness. I am committed to making sure I get enough sleep because I know how bad I feel when I do not.

Throughout the first fifteen years of my running career, I never struggled with injuries to the extent I have over the last three years. In 2013, on my fortieth birthday, I went out for a twenty-two-mile run and experienced a cramp on the bottom of my foot. I finally had to admit my foot was not getting better and went to a doctor, who told me I had torn my plantar fascia. I took six months off of running and started swimming to stay in cardiovascular shape.

Then, a week before my forty-first birthday, I felt pain in my other foot. The pain became so intense that I would become nauseated and start sweating if I accidentally put my heel on the ground. At first my doctor thought it was a stress fracture, but four months later I was still on crutches and had not seen any improvement. I finally saw a different doctor, who discovered I had ruptured my other plantar fascia and entrapped a nerve. He said my case was so severe that he would consider doing surgery immediately, but he told me to go home and think about what I wanted to do. I told him I did not need to think about it at all. I was ready to be able to walk again and would do anything to get better.

After the surgery, I was walking again within a month but felt a sudden pop on the top of my foot. I ended up with a stress fracture, which is a rare side effect of the surgery but was due more to the fact that I was walking for the first time in seven months. Much to my frustration, I was back on crutches for three more months. It is mind-blowing to think that I went from running several marathons each year to being injured for two solid years and on crutches for almost half of that.

I worked to come back very slowly and finally entered my first post-injury race in December 2015. I was absolutely thrilled to cross the finish line because I had been living with a nagging fear that I may never be able to run again. During my time off I entered several swim meets and even finished 5K and 10K swim competitions in the Cayman Islands. I found that the swimming kept me fit and distracted me from running. However, my first love will always be running, especially at Memorial Park. Even when I was on crutches with my foot injuries, I would come to the Park and crutch around the trail. It is a great oasis in the middle of our city.

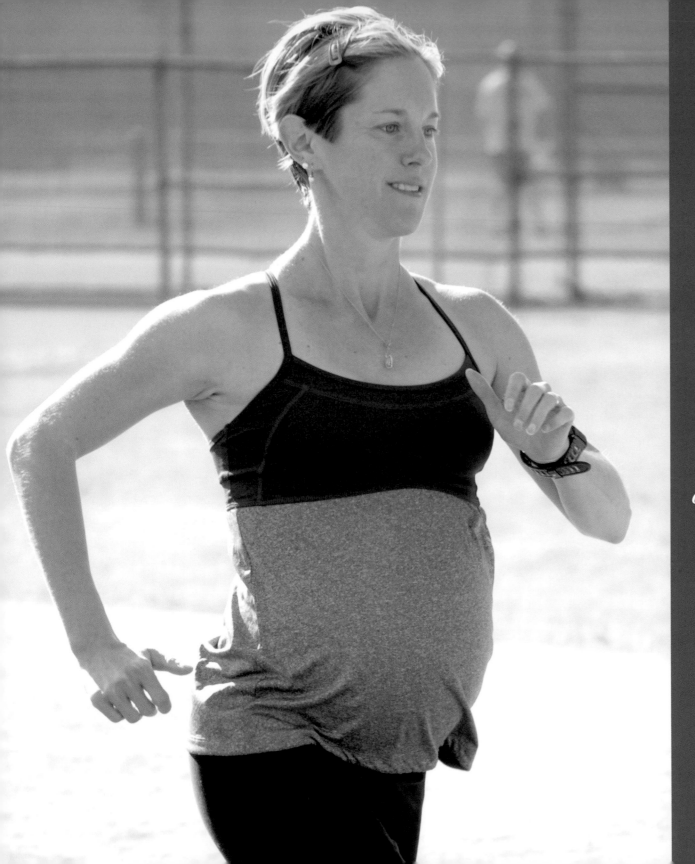

When I was thirty-five weeks pregnant, I had a friend ask me to help her get through the last eight miles of her long run, even though I was only planning to run six easy miles. Of course I said, "Sure! Why not? I can do that with you!"

CHRISTY LAN

I grew up in Louisville, Kentucky, and was active as a child but never ran. During my last two years of engineering school, a friend and I decided to incorporate quick jogging breaks into our study sessions as a way to relieve stress. Over the next two years, especially during finals, we continued to jog as a way to clear our brains. We never ran more than a mile, but I always felt much better and could think more clearly when I sat back down to continue plowing through the material.

After I graduated from college, I took a job in New Orleans. The company I worked for asked me to fill out a get-to-know-you questionnaire, and I checked a box that said I enjoyed being outdoors. A couple of coworkers saw my information and invited me to participate in a 5K mud run. Even though I had said I liked being outdoors, I insisted there was no way I could run that far. They convinced me I would have fun eating lunch at a bar after the race, so I agreed to sign up.

I was excited to meet many people that day, but several of them said they were training for an Ironman triathlon, which I had never heard of. When they told me how far they planned to race, I thought they were absolutely crazy. They invited me to join them for dinner on Wednesday nights after their normal triathlon training sessions. A few weeks later, a couple of girls in the group convinced me to show up an hour earlier and run two miles with them. At first I tried to argue that I could not possibly keep up with someone who was training for an Ironman, but they insisted, and I finally agreed. I should have known where it would lead, but a few months later, they also convinced me to buy a bike. Before I knew it, I was signing up for a triathlon, which was the most ridiculous thing I could have imagined a year earlier. The improvements in my fitness over those two years were impressive, but more than anything I loved being with my friends.

When Hurricane Katrina hit New Orleans in August 2005, I was transferred to Houston. One of my friends who had moved from New Orleans to Houston the year before met a guy who was also a runner and biker, and he offered to help us find the best places to exercise in Houston. I told him I preferred to work out at 5:00 a.m. but was nervous about running by myself, so he volunteered to meet me at Memorial Park three days per week. At the time I did not realize that he did not normally exercise in the morning. After we began dating, he admitted that he did not enjoy waking up at 4:30 a.m. and usually ran at night.

After our son was born in 2014, we decided to alternate days for who gets to exercise outside. I run at the Park on Tuesdays, Thursdays, and Saturdays. When it is my turn to stay home, I turn the baby monitor on and ride a trainer in our garage apartment. I rarely get to exercise with my husband now, but our priorities have shifted, and we know it is more important to spend time together as a family.

During my first pregnancy, I had a friend who was also expecting. We exercised together and decided to see if we could set personal records for the marathon after our babies were born. At first we tried to train for the Portland Marathon, which would have given us ten months to get in shape. However, a couple months before the race, we realized that we needed more time. We ended up flying to Portland and running for fun but also decided to sign up for the Houston Marathon, which was a couple months later. To my delight, in January 2015 (one year after I had my son) I ran the marathon in three hours, thirteen minutes—a four-minute improvement on my personal record.

Because I raced so well in Houston, I decided to sign up for Ironman Texas. I promised my husband that I would maintain the same schedule we already had in place. There was one weekend when my friends came in town, and I trained really hard for the entire weekend, but besides that, I wanted to make sure my family was still the main priority, regardless of the race. I have every other Friday off from work, so I would get on the trainer at 4:30 a.m. and ride for two hours. Then I would take my son to school and drive to Katy, where I would ride for four more hours. I was grateful to get in six-hour bike rides, even if I did have to take a two-hour break in the middle of the workout.

The best thing about all this training was that it did not take time away from my family. I did have to start waking up at 4:00 instead of 4:30, but it was all worth it. I was performing at the same level or even better than I had before my son was born. I just had to focus and train harder with the limited time I had.

I love running, but I go to Memorial Park because I want to start my day with people I enjoy being around. Running at the Park is my social time. I love the conversations with my friends and catching up on their lives. If it means I have to wake up twenty minutes earlier to drive to the Park, I don't mind because it makes the start to my day fun. It is also the only time during the day when I can be my own person. I am not mom, wife, or employee. It is extremely therapeutic to have my own time, even if it is just an hour.

Many people do not realize how crowded the Park is in the early mornings. After I had my son, I was hesitant to move my start time up from 5:00 a.m., but I quickly realized there is always someone I know at the Park, even at 4:30 in the morning. Another interesting aspect of the Park is that there are people whom I consider "friends" even though we have never formally met. We just wave at each other. For someone who has never been to Memorial Park, it is hard to understand.

After my son was born, I thought about hiring a coach. Then my husband asked what I would do if the coach scheduled a certain workout but my friends all said they were going to do something totally different. He was right; he knows me. Why pay a coach when I would not follow his schedule if my friends were doing something else?

I was really worried when I got pregnant for the second time because I thought I was going to have to run by myself for nine months. However, it ended up being the biggest blessing. I started working out with a few people who ran with a different pace group, and I quickly developed some very strong friendships.

It was also perfect timing because they were all starting to train for the Houston Marathon. Because I was comfortable running at their pace, I got to be their cheerleader. I loved being able to encourage them when they were not feeling well and helping them push through the tough days. When I was thirty-five weeks pregnant, a friend asked me to help her get through the last eight miles of her long run, even though I was only planning to run six easy miles that morning. Of course I said, "Sure! Why not? I can do that with you!" I treasure the lasting friendships I have made and am excited to return to the Park as soon as I recover from having my second son.

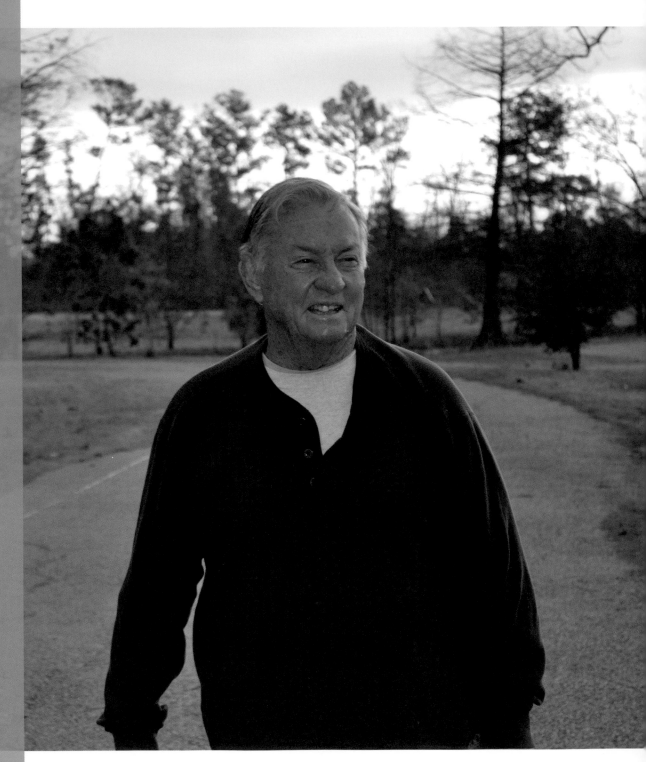

The planning and construction of a quarter-mile track at Memorial Park was a peculiar thing. In the end, Roy Cullen and I agreed it was better to have a three-lane track than a no-lane track.

AL LAWRENCE

As a young man, I was a world-class runner in Australia. One thing I am renowned for is giving everyone I meet a nickname. This is because the society I grew up in was originally full of convicts. They spoke in codes so the prison guards would not understand what they were talking about. This manner of communicating carried over to my generation, where almost everyone and everything had a nickname.

If someone did not know the group of kids I grew up with, he would think we were terrible to each other! Most of my friends had names that described the shape of their heads or the size of their brains. There was Boof Head, Block Head, Pumpkin Head, Egg Head, Chizzle Head, Cement Head, and the Village Idiot. My name was given not because of my head but because of my weight. As a teenager, I was extremely thin. My friends started calling me Fat Al, which was quickly shortened to Fat. Even when I went back to Australia after graduating from the University of Houston, my friends were constantly saying, "Fat! Where have you been?"

I won a bronze medal for the ten thousand meters in the 1956 Olympics and set the world record for the indoor two mile in 1960. Two years after I graduated from UH, I became the assistant track and cross-country coach. I also started working on the side, coaching individuals throughout Houston. Occasionally we would run at Memorial Park because it was a central place to meet, but there was only a worn dirt path in the early days. The City eventually scraped the dirt and laid a trail of wood chips. There were places along the loop where my feet sank down and the wood chips covered my ankles.

Although I enjoyed coaching some of Houston's finest runners for several years, I also needed the security of a reliable paycheck. I was hired to be the general manager of a small audiovisual company, but many clients and friends continued to encourage me to quit my full-time job and become a professional coach.

Then one evening I received an invitation to have dinner at the home of my longtime clients and friends, Roy and Mary Cullen. We discussed my dilemma, and Roy offered to hire me as the coach of the Cullen family for the next eighteen months. He said he would pay me a monthly stipend for my services to give me time to develop my client base. As I drove home from dinner with the Cullens, I realized that not only had I just been offered my dream job, but I was also going to be paid more than I had ever imagined—at least for the next eighteen months. The next day, I turned in my two weeks' notice and embarked on my new career.

By the early 1980s, I was coaching a large group of runners, and we were meeting at Lamar or Memorial High School for the track workouts. However, we were at the mercy of the schools. If they ever had something else going on, we would have to find another place to run or change the workout. One afternoon, Roy and I were discussing how it was a crying shame we were in the fourth-largest city in the United States but did not have a public track. The planning and construction of a quarter-mile track at Memorial Park was a peculiar thing, but Roy agreed to finance the construction if I could find a place to put it.

At that time, the "tree-hugger" movement was in full swing, and Houstonians were going to great lengths to avoid cutting down trees. I scouted various spots around the Park, but there were enormous trees everywhere. I asked a local engineer to help me with a few design concepts and was finally able to lay out a regulation, 440-yard, linear track. It was a soft, all-purpose, six-lane track and fit perfectly between the road in front of the Tennis Center and Katy Freeway. Roy paid for the engineering drawings, and I excitedly carried them to the Houston Parks Department.

The City examined my drawings and informed me that they had plans to add parking along the street in front of the Tennis Center. Also, they were planning to build concrete berms that would minimize the noise adjacent to the Katy Freeway. Finally, the Corps of Engineers had designated the muddy area in the middle of my design as a navigable waterway. The track could not encroach upon this federally protected channel. After all of the trouble I had put myself through to avoid tearing down all but one bloody tree, it would have been nice to have known this from the beginning!

My plan was ditched, but I was told I could resubmit a new plan as long as the design fit within their restrictions. I talked to Roy and told him that in order to meet the City's requests, the track would have to be a weird configuration, but I felt like it was our only option. We agreed it was better to have a three-lane track than a no-lane track.

I was at the Park in 1987 when they finally poured the surface. The surveyor's stakes look like small nails and can still be seen at each 110 mark. I ran the first quarter mile as soon as they finished painting the lines. Since then, I have coached thousands of runners and spent countless hours at that track—it is my second home.

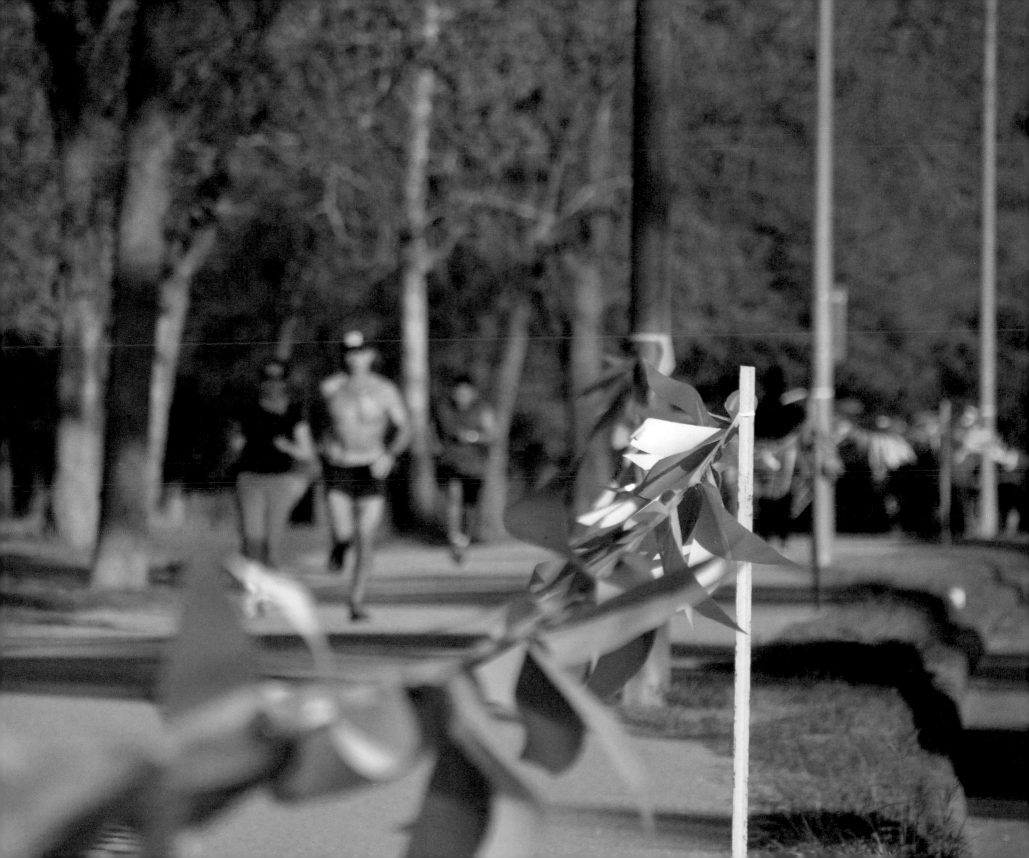

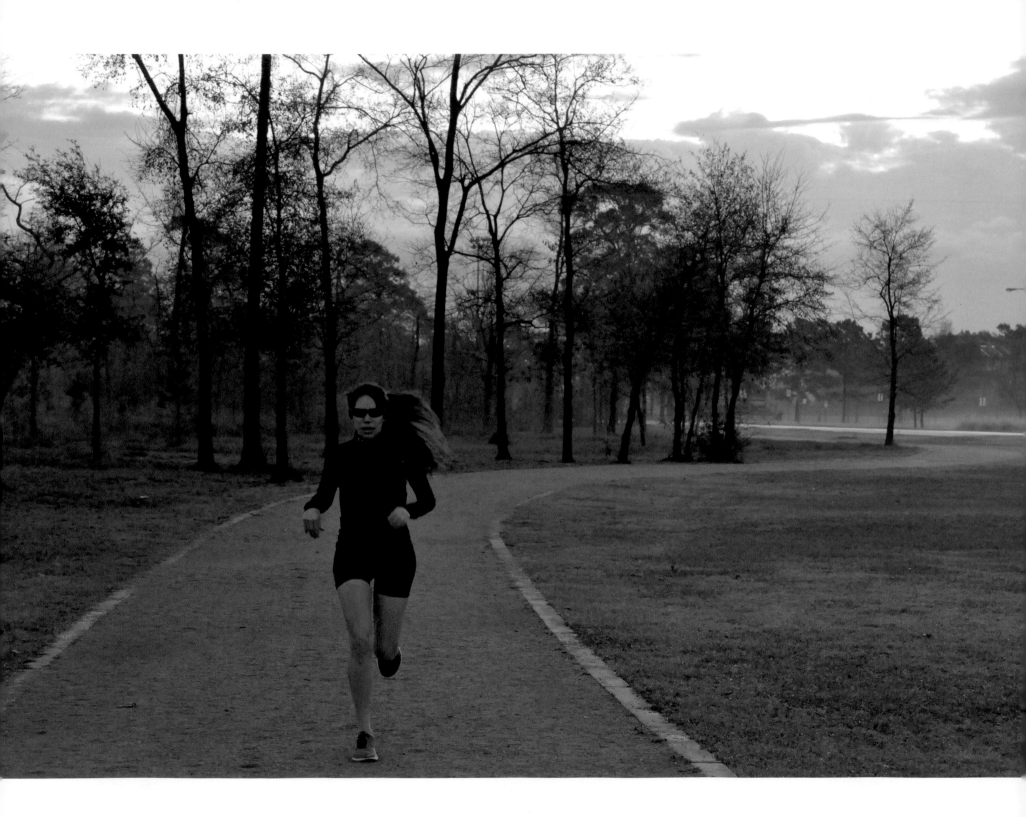

MARI McCAIN

I was born in Peru and moved to Houston in 1992 to attend college. After I started running, I heard that Coach Jim McLatchie could help me improve my times. To my surprise, when I went to meet him, he said I was too slow and he was not interested in coaching me. He told me to get my 5K time under twenty minutes and then write him a letter about why I wanted to run for him. I worked hard to improve and finally broke twenty minutes. Then, in the letter, I said that I may not be the fastest, but I wanted to get better. I told him I had a passion for running. I do not know if he even read the letter, but he did finally agree to coach me.

In 2010, shortly after I turned thirty-five, I began feeling exhausted during my easy runs and was frustrated because my times were getting slower. I went to the doctor and was told my iron level was low. After a couple months of iron supplements, my levels rose, but I still felt tired and nauseated. Finally, my doctor suggested I take a pregnancy test. To my shock, I was almost five months pregnant! My husband and I had watched a show on television about women who had babies and never knew they were pregnant. We used to laugh at those girls, but all of the sudden I realized I was one of them!

Today, I run at Memorial Park at least two times each week. I live in Katy, which is forty-five minutes away, but I do not mind the drive. Over the last twenty years, there are many people I have met at the Park. Although we do not do anything together outside of running, I still consider them some of my best friends.

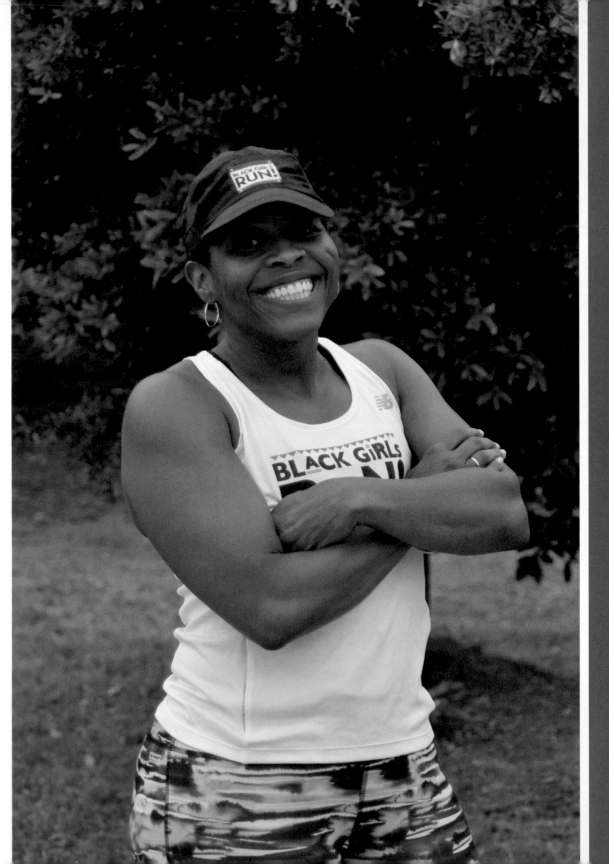

I stared at the photo thinking, Is that really me? I knew I had to make a change, and after a year of running with BGR and teaching dance and fitness classes, I had lost ninety pounds.

XAVI McDUELL
& BLACK GIRLS RUN!

When I was in the seventh grade I joined my middle school cross-country team, and our first meet was held along Allen Parkway. A quarter mile into the race, I seriously thought, *I am going to die*. At that point I decided I was never, ever going to run again. I was a cheerleader in high school and planned to cheer in college but got pregnant with my daughter. I had my son four years later, and after both pregnancies, I quickly lost the weight and dropped back down to my previous size.

For the next fifteen years, I maintained a schedule of regularly going to the gym after work, but then I got depressed and stopped exercising for a while. My weight slowly started creeping up, so I joined Weight Watchers and resolved to wake up every morning and walk five miles. I ended up losing thirty-five pounds in three months! After I lost the weight, I stopped walking but continued going to the gym and eating well.

In 2013, I got depressed again and found myself in the same place I was before. One day I was in my kindergarten schoolroom passing out our class picture and was shocked when I actually took the time to look at the photo. There I was standing next to my kids, but I had gained so much weight that I did not recognize myself. I stared at the photo thinking, *Is that really me?* The next thing I knew, I was mad at everyone in the world who had not been truthful enough to tell me I was fat! My daughter even tried to encourage me by saying I was just wearing an unflattering shirt, but I knew I had to make a change.

I had a friend who was constantly posting on Facebook about how she was a member of Black Girls RUN! (BGR) and loved exercising with the group. In the back of my mind, every time I saw her posts I would think about that middle school cross-country meet. It scarred me for life. Finally I decided I had to give it a try. I joined BGR and started following a Couch to 5K schedule.

Shortly after I began working out with the group, another girl and I were jogging together in my neighborhood. I told myself that even though I was exhausted, I was going to keep running until she stopped. I kept looking at her, waiting for her to stop, but she just kept going. To my surprise, we ended up doing three miles without walking! As we were catching our breath, she said, "Girl, if you had not kept running, I would have stopped a long time ago! Thanks for keeping me going!" Then of course I had to laugh, because the only reason I had run the entire thing was because I was watching her. That experience showed me how important belonging to a club like BGR can be. We motivated each other, which is exactly what I needed.

Because Houston is such a big city, BGR is divided into ten regions. A city-wide run is held at Memorial Park on the first Saturday of every month, and members meet within their regions throughout the month. In May 2013, I attended my first city-wide run. Before that time, I had a friend who talked about going to Memorial Park, but I thought he was crazy to drive all that way to run. In addition to finally being able to meet the other BGR members from across the city, I loved everything about the Park: the trees, the people, and the excitement of exercising with such a big group. Since that first city-wide run three years ago, I have attended almost every meeting.

That summer I signed up for my first race, a five-mile run that was being held on the same day as a ten-mile race. I knew I could do three miles and thought I would have time to build up enough strength for the longer race. A couple weeks before the event, I was looking at the race website and saw that the ten-mile finishers would receive a medal, but the five-mile participants did not get anything. I did not want to do a race if I was not going to get a medal, so at the last minute I switched to the longer distance, even though I had never run more than three miles. In September 2013, I was thrilled to finally finish my first race, which was ten times longer than the middle school cross-country meet thirty years earlier.

During this time, I also went back to the gym and started taking a Soul Grooves class. I decided to get certified to teach Soul Grooves, RIPPED, and Zumba, because I love dancing and was excited that I could actually get paid to do it! As soon as I became certified, my evenings filled up teaching classes across the city. By March 2014, after a year of being with BGR and teaching dance and fitness classes, I had lost ninety pounds.

In 2015, I applied to be the Houston ambassador for BGR. Although it is a volunteer position, the parent organization in Atlanta takes it very seriously. They want to make sure I am dedicated to the organization and can represent them well. During the group runs, I am not there to get my own workout in. Instead, I encourage everyone and work to make sure they have a good experience. Before each city-wide run, I give announcements and tell the group that no one is going to get left behind. It does not matter who is last, I will always stay with her. When I started running in 2013, my biggest concern was that I was going to slow everyone down, but the national motto is "No Girl Left Behind." I like to add "Your Race, Your Pace." When someone starts running for the first time, she usually tries to take off sprinting, but I think it is better to encourage her to go slow and just make sure she can finish. We can work on the speed later.

Today, in addition to being a kindergarten teacher and ambassador for BGR, I also teach ten classes at gyms throughout Houston each week. Just as I see children mature and grow in the classroom, I am also amazed at how many people I have touched through running and exercise. Sometimes I wonder where I would be if I had worked out seriously when I was younger. I regret that I started so late in life, but the changes I have seen in myself and the BGR members over the last three years have been tremendously rewarding.

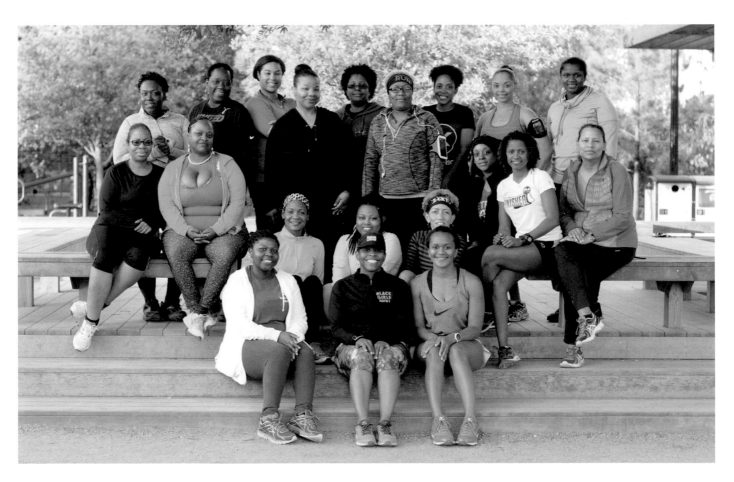

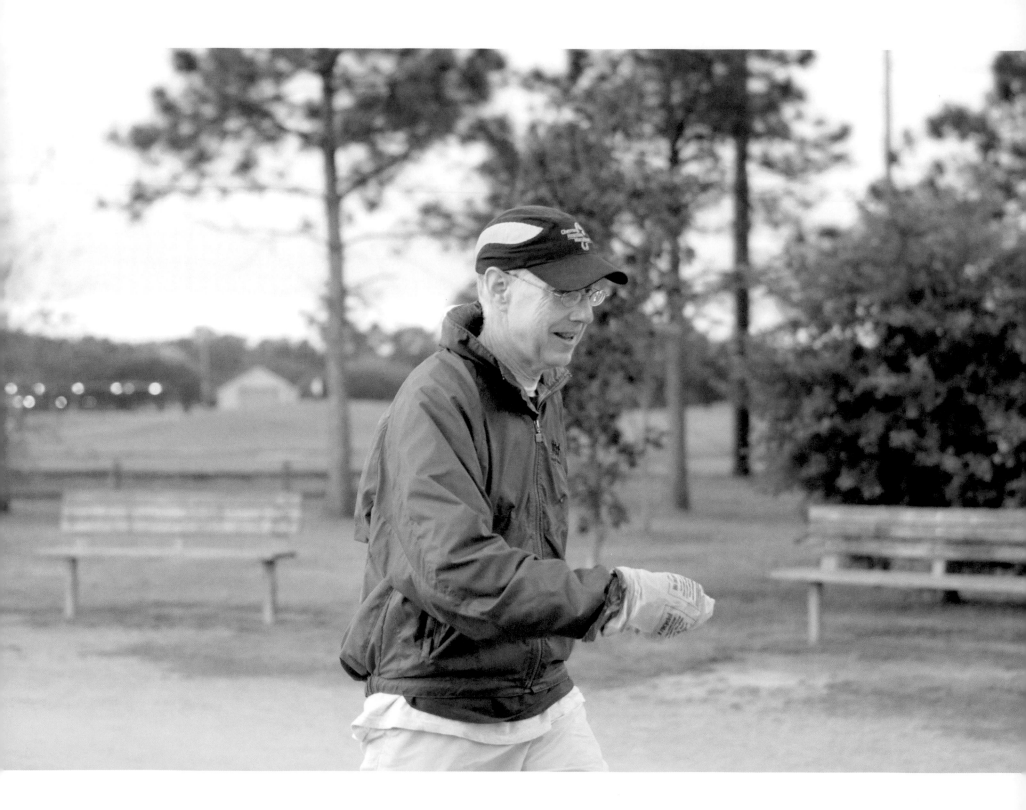

MARK MUCH

I walk at Memorial Park every morning. A couple years ago, after my dog died, I realized I still had several hundred plastic bags in my home. I decided to bring them to the Park and pick up trash as I made my way around the trail. I eventually ran out of the doggie bags, so now I just use plastic, newspaper, or grocery bags.

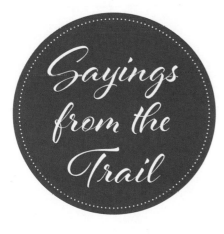

"Do you want to stay up or go down?"

There is a ten-mile out-and-back route that leaves the Park and follows Buffalo Bayou before returning to the Park. The Bayou portion of the route has two main paths, one of which has many hills. Houston's runners are used to flat roads, so some people prefer to avoid the dips of the lower route and run along the top.

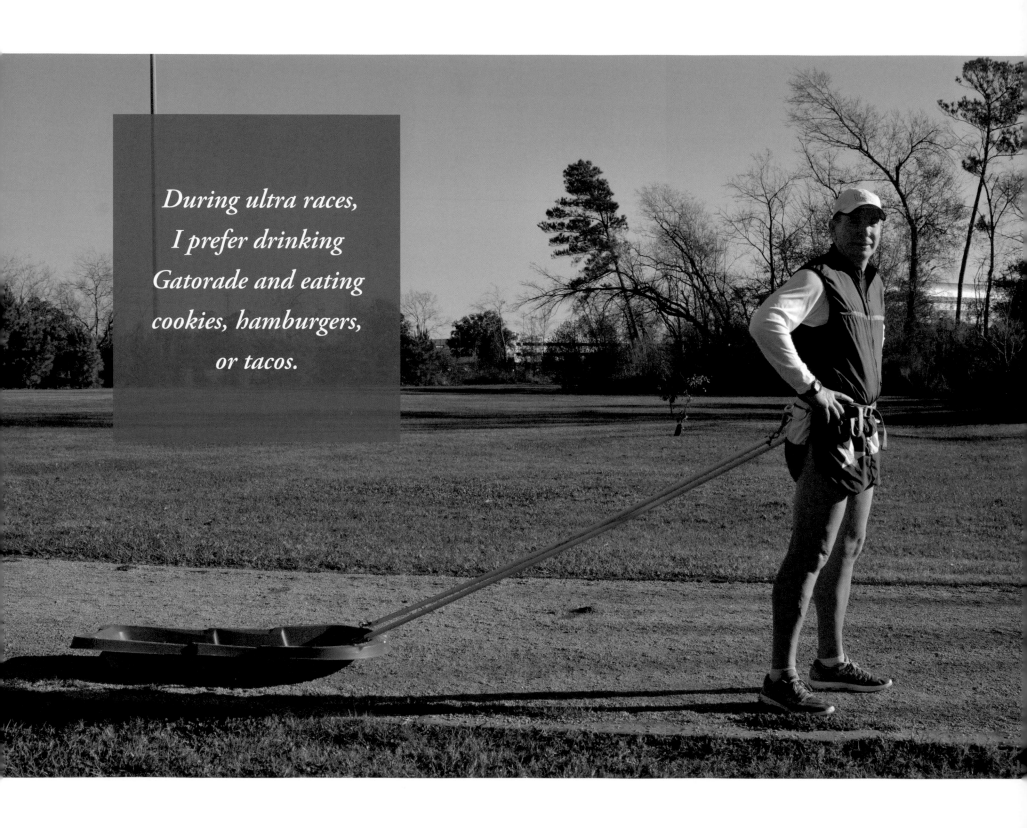

During ultra races,
I prefer drinking
Gatorade and eating
cookies, hamburgers,
or tacos.

TIM NECKAR

I grew up in Arizona and began running when I was thirteen years old. I visited Houston a couple times before it became my home in 1992. During those trips, I would run at Memorial Park because it was a convenient place to get my workouts in while traveling. However, my primary thought after exercising at the Park was, *Who wants to run in a three-mile loop?*

After I moved to Houston, I was looking for a way to earn additional income. I liked the thought of personal training but knew I did not want to be stuck in a gym. I decided it would be a perfect fit if I combined coaching and running. In 1995, I started my business, runnerOne, which not only provides my clients with workout schedules but also accompanies them stride-for-stride during their workouts.

Despite my initial hesitations about running in a three-mile loop, I quickly realized the Park was the perfect place to be seen. So I printed one thousand flyers and put them on cars that were parked near the Tennis Center. I only received one response, but over the past twenty years, I have gradually expanded my business.

On weekdays, I schedule two coaching sessions in the mornings starting at 5:00 a.m., and then I go to T.H. Rogers Middle School, where I teach PE. After school is out, I go back to the Park to run with two or three more clients. I also meet my athletes on Sunday mornings, but on Saturdays, I run by myself and spend time away from the Park.

A few of my clients have also asked me to pace them during races, which I enjoy because it gives us a change in scenery. In 2016, one of my athletes wanted to know if she could bring my wife and me to Paris so I could accompany her during the Paris Marathon. I told her that even though it would be a tough assignment, I guessed I was up for it. It was a wonderful experience and just another reason why I love my job.

My career as a middle school PE teacher resembles my life as the owner of runnerOne. At school, the class period is very structured, and the kids know they are coming to the gym to exercise and not just play. However, I like to say we have "serious fun," because the kids need a way to relieve stress and get a quality workout at the same time.

I strive to log at least three thousand miles per year and am almost always training for an upcoming ultramarathon. I lift weights and rotate through about twelve different pairs of shoes per week. I also think running on the softer surface at the Park and training at various speeds has helped me avoid injuries.

A couple of my favorite events are the Rim to Rim to Rim run, which travels from one side of the Grand Canyon to the other and back again, and the 126.2-mile Rouge Orleans race, which I won by over three hours in 2015. I maintain an old-school philosophy regarding hydration and fueling during longer races. I prefer drinking Gatorade and eating cookies, hamburgers, or tacos during ultra runs. I have never tried the newer gels or bars. I know what works, so I do not see any reason to change.

Besides the numerous hours per week I spend with my clients, some people at the Park may remember me better as the man who could be seen dragging a plastic sled around the trail. This was part of my training for the 135-mile Arrowhead Ultra race in Minnesota in which the competitors are required to carry their own gear and support equipment. The sled glided across the crushed granite at the Park similar to the way it moved across the snow in Minnesota. I put a fifty-pound weight in the sled, which was similar to the weight of the items I had to pull during the race.

One year, around Christmas time, I thought it would be fun to also attach lights and tinsel to the sled. However, I did not need the decorations to attract attention. Everyone on the trail knew when I was getting close to them because they could hear the sled dragging across the ground from a long way off.

I work with a wide range of athletes, from those who are starting to run for the first time in their lives to others who have been competing for years and are trying to set new personal records. I am skilled at maintaining any pace between six and thirteen minutes per mile. I'm sure my ability to pace my clients is enhanced by the miles I have accumulated during my life. I completed my first marathon when I was fourteen years old and have never looked back.

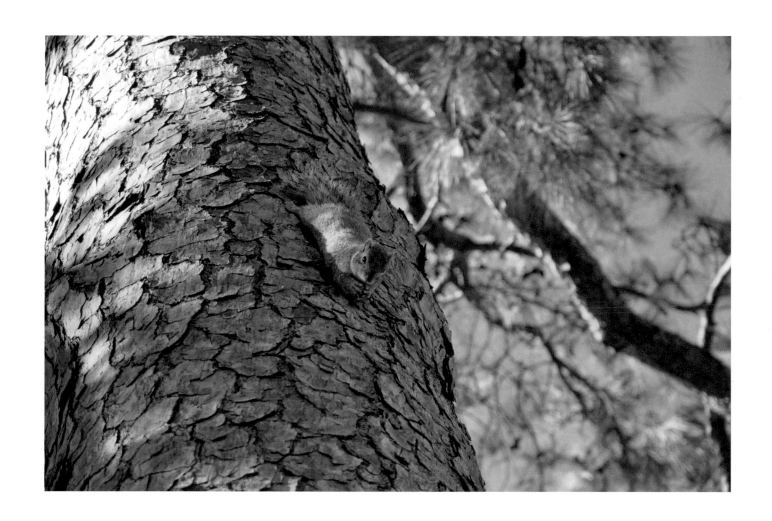

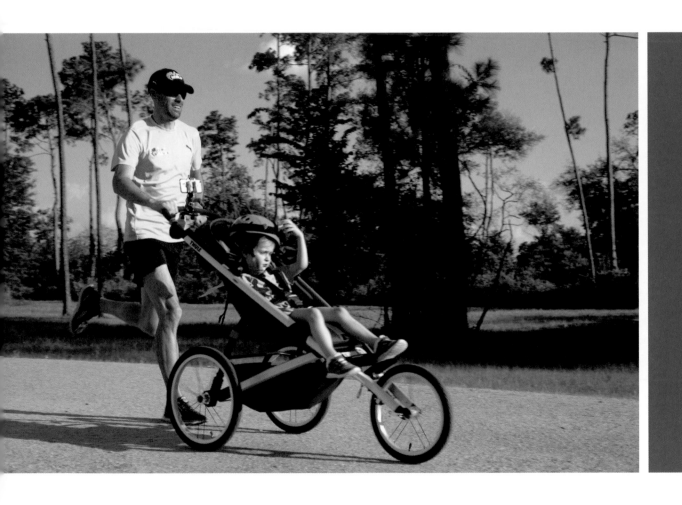

*In February 2016,
my youngest daughter
and I set the world record
for the fastest half marathon
while pushing a stroller.*

CALUM NEFF

*I*ran at Memorial Park for the first time when I was competing for the University of Houston. My teammates and I would zoom around the trail, and I miss being able to train in a big pack like that. When I was in college, I thought I was very mature and fit, but today, when I see the team running at the Park, I think they all look young and skinny.

I am looking forward to the next phase of the Park, which is supposed to include a new quarter-mile track. Houston really needs a public track for people like me who want to train hard. I also enjoy running on the trails on the south side of the Park. They help to cure my itch to go trail running.

In February 2016, my youngest daughter and I set the world record for the fastest half marathon while pushing a stroller. We finished in one hour, eleven minutes, and twenty-seven seconds, averaging five minutes, twenty-seven seconds per mile. I began running with the stroller in 2012, after my oldest daughter was born. We lived a couple miles away from the Park, and I would bring a speaker that blared music so people could hear us coming and get out of our way. The publicity and excitement following our world-record race was incredible, and I never imagined it would be that well received. The feedback has actually given me a purpose for running. I want to encourage others to find their passions while maintaining balance with their families.

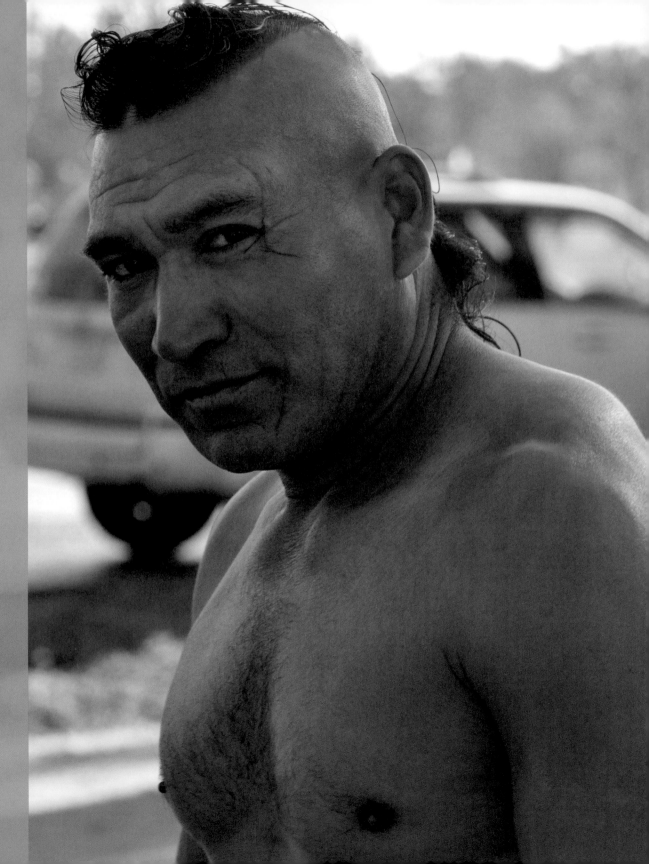

A member of the Tornados Running Club approached me and asked why I was running in jeans, cowboy boots, and a button-down flannel shirt. He loaned me a pair of "real" running shoes and invited me to ride with him to Memorial Park.

FRANCISCO PEREZ

I was raised in the mountains of Mexico where there is a rich Indian history. People often ask me what happened to cause the scar on my face, but I would rather tell the story of the scar they cannot see that streaks across my foot. The events that occurred after that horrific accident changed my life in a way I could have never imagined but were all for the better.

The culture I grew up in placed a high value on hard, physical labor, dedication to the family, and enduring hardship for the sake of a better life. I came to the United States seeking a way to provide for my family and escape the brutal sufferings of my hometown. Even though I did not have any formal education or training, I was fortunate to find a job working on a farm mowing grass.

As I was driving the mower, a pin that held the trailer in alignment fell out and could not be located. In order to get the job done in a timely manner, I decided to replace the missing pin with a screwdriver. It didn't take long for the mower to start having problems again, so I put the vehicle in park and hopped off to take a look.

To my shock, the screwdriver had fallen out and the mower was moving forward on its own. It began shredding the top of my foot, and my coworkers at the farm rushed me to the emergency room where I was immediately admitted for surgery. The rapid loss of blood almost ended my life, but the doctors were miraculously able to stop the bleeding and stitch my damaged tendons and bones together.

When I was discharged from the hospital, the doctor advised me to keep my foot moving in order to regain flexibility. Although I had never run before, I decided to visit Mason Park, on the southeast side of Houston, where I had recently noticed people exercising. Over the next couple weeks, I built up enough strength to complete several laps around Mason Park each evening.

One day, a member of the Tornados Running Club approached me and asked why I was running in jeans, cowboy boots, and a button-down flannel shirt. I told him I was just following my doctor's orders in an attempt to rehabilitate my injured foot. He loaned me a pair of "real" running shoes and invited me to ride with him to Memorial Park.

A few days later, as I ran at the Park for the first time in my life, I felt like a new person. It was not only the new running shoes but also the feeling of the wind against my face and the spring in my step. I was convinced I could fly.

My friend began driving me to the Park on a regular basis, and I was fortunate enough to meet several other members of the Tornados Running Club. I was surprised at how they included me in their workouts and encouraged me when I was tired. Slowly, over the next few years, I began to enter fun runs and was proud that I won or placed at the top of my age group despite only having been running for a short time.

As I look back and think about my circumstances when I first moved to Houston, I am overwhelmed at what I have become and the tremendous influence my friends at the Park have had on my life. There was a time in the late 1990s when my wife, who was nine months pregnant, fell and was in severe pain. One of the Tornados members was an ultrasound technician and offered to let my wife visit the doctor's office for free. We did not know if the baby had survived the fall but were thrilled to hear its heart still beating a few days later. Shortly after the ultrasound, the Tornados threw a surprise baby shower and inundated us with gifts for our new arrival.

That same baby is now a teenager. In the spring of 2016, he was diagnosed with cancer and lost all of his hair while undergoing chemotherapy treatments. I am brought to tears as I watch my son endure such terrible conditions, but once again the Tornados have rallied to provide financial assistance during these hard times. I am thankful for their never-ending support and encouragement, not only to me but also to my family.

Although many people at the Park do not know my story, they recognize my unique haircut and running form. I like to shave my hair in a Mohawk because I want to be different and believe I should honor my Indian heritage. Occasionally, when I am feeling daring, I will also shave lines down the sides of my head.

However, my desire to stand out and look different is not really necessary when I hit the trail at the Park. I turned fifty in 2012 but can still keep up with my friends, who are half my age. Today, I am thankful to be alive and able to drive to the Park on my own. If my friend had not loaned me a pair of running shoes, I might still be jogging around Mason Park in my boots!

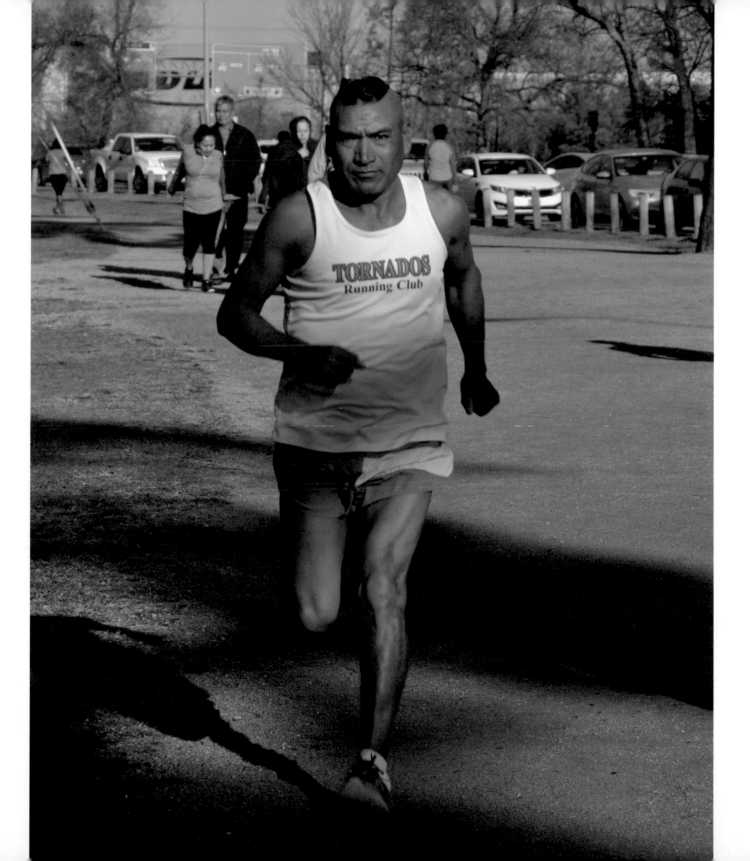

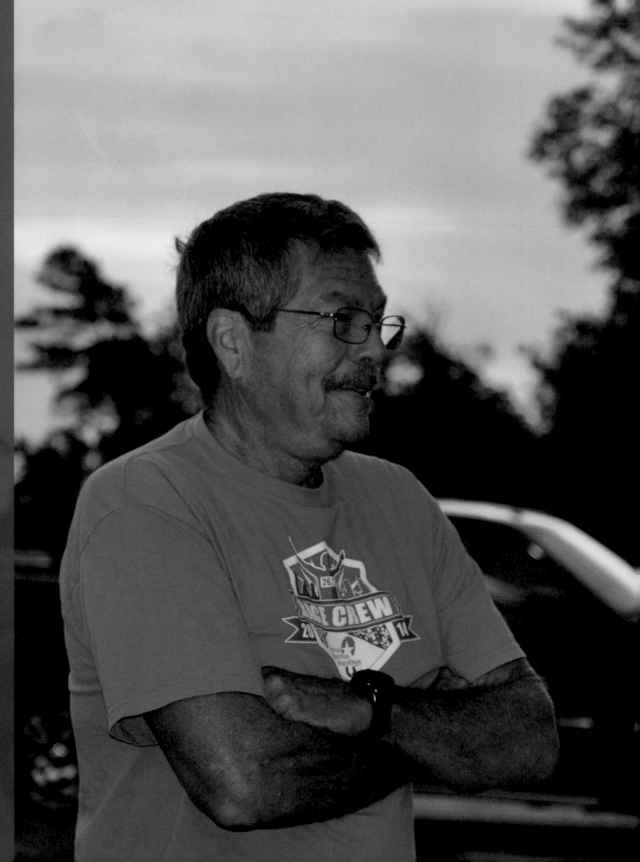

I relished the idea of belonging to a team and working to achieve a common goal. I was the first person in Houston to bring a portable tent to a fun run. Besides the tent, I also bring a toilet to all the club races.

JOHN PHILLIPS

I moved to Houston in 1975 after reading that the climate was one of the best in the country for waterskiing year-round. I was twenty-five years old, did not have a job, and did not know anyone, but waterskiing was my passion.

One Friday morning in 1986, I was reading the newspaper and saw that a marathon was coming to town that Sunday. Since I did not have anything else going on that weekend, I decided I would try it even though I had never run a step in my life. The only thing that kept me going during the race was not knowing that walking was allowed. I ran the whole way because I thought I would be disqualified if I stopped. I already had a commitment to go bowling with my friends that night and did not want to back out. Somehow I managed to bowl, but I could not stand up straight for the next two days.

The following year, I was reading the newspaper again and saw the damn thing was coming back to Houston in two weeks. Even though I had not run a step in the previous fifty weeks, I was excited, because this time I actually had a chance to train! I decided to run four miles in the morning and four more at night every day for the two weeks leading up to the event. The training worked, and I dropped fifteen minutes off my time from the previous year. Once again, I thought the rules required me to run the entire thing. Now, thirty years later, I have completed seventy marathons, including twenty-four Houston Marathons.

During that second race, I realized that Houston had a huge running community. I even saw a couple of people I knew. They invited me to meet them on Sunday mornings at Memorial Park for a long run. A few years later, I joined the Bayou City Road Runners (BCRR) club. I relished the idea of belonging to a team and working to achieve a common goal. I was president of BCRR from 1996 to 1999 and am proud that the membership grew from forty people to 250 in that short time. I told the other members who wanted to run with me that they could come to the Park on Sunday mornings. That tradition still stands today. Sometimes we have as many as fifty people who show up.

I was the first person in Houston to bring a portable tent to a fun run. Shortly after I became president of BCRR, I noticed that most of the runners milled around after races, and it was difficult to find everyone. I told the club I had a surprise I was planning to bring to the next event. Just as I began to set the tent up, a race organizer stormed up and insisted I take it down. A brief argument ensued, but by the time the race was over, we were all standing under our tent. Most of the other running clubs also have tents now, but we were the first.

In 1997, the club organized a beach run in which everyone ran in Galveston and then had a party on the sand. Our problem was that there were not any public restrooms close to the beach. The following year I told everyone I had another surprise. I used some leftover material from my construction business and built a portable toilet. I hoisted the toilet on my trailer and drove it down to Galveston. The club members cheered when they saw me rolling up with an outhouse. Besides the tent, I also now bring the toilet to all the club races. I have to be the Porta-Potty Policeman because people try to sneak in and use it. I tell them if they pee now they can pay later because they will have to join the club.

I am also a stickler for being on time. I feel like I have trained the club to respect the fact that when we say we are going to start running from the Park at 6:30 a.m., we mean it. I tell people that if they show up at the Tennis Center at 6:31, they won't see a soul. I learned that if we became relaxed, then pretty soon we were starting at 7:00. Also, I like to see the club start as a group. It shows we value our team and stick together. Over the years, the cohesiveness of our club can also be seen in the ten marriages between members. Most of those relationships started at the Park during a Sunday morning long run.

In 2001, I decided to hold a twenty-one-mile long run from my house a few weeks before the Houston Marathon. It was an easy excuse to have a big party. I called it John's Looooooong Run. I laid out the course, which meandered through Memorial Park, River Oaks, and Tanglewood and then headed back to my house. Then I walked the entire route with a survey wheel so I could measure and plot the exact point of each mile. It took me three days to certify the course. When I was racing, I always became upset if I passed the one-mile marker five minutes into the race, which I knew was impossible. There are many other runners who are just like me; we want to know "a mile" is a mile. Since that first Looooooong Run fifteen years ago, I have gone back every year to spray-paint the mile markers so they are easily seen.

While everyone is out on the course, I stay home with a few volunteers and cook a huge breakfast with a lot of bacon. My wife, however, has always hated the smell of bacon. She was also not too fond of seeing the sweaty runners walking around our home and reclining on our couches. After the first couple years, she announced that she was leaving the house on the morning of the run but that when she returned that afternoon, the house had better pass inspection. In 2013, we had ninety-five people who participated in John's Loooooong Run. I spent hours on my knees mopping up puddles of sweat and trying my best to get rid of the bacon smell. The following year, I finally broke down and agreed to make everyone stay outside on our driveway. I also agreed to cook the bacon in the garage so the smell would not permeate our bedrooms. To my delight, my wife agreed to stay home and help with the party!

Although running has generally kept me healthy, in 2013 I noticed a lump in my neck. After numerous tests, I was told it was cancer. I went through several weeks of chemo and radiation and had to endure a feeding tube for seven months. The entire experience left me exhausted. I own my business, so I decided to take a year off of work and focus on getting through the treatments. In my twenty-five years of running before the cancer, I never wore a shirt, regardless of the temperature. Many people at the Park thought I was nuts when they would see me in freezing weather, but I was very warm-blooded. Since my battle with cancer, I have often found myself looking for a jacket and feeling cold.

The cancer also left me less motivated to run. I have found it difficult to get back into running given the dramatic changes that occurred in my body. However, even though I have not personally completed a Memorial Park long run in a couple years, I can still be found at the Park every Sunday morning. I see the other club members off on their run. Then I drive to the River Oaks Rose Garden, where I talk to everyone as they stop for a drink. I still find satisfaction in seeing the members of our club succeed and am happy to support them, regardless of my personal exercise routine.

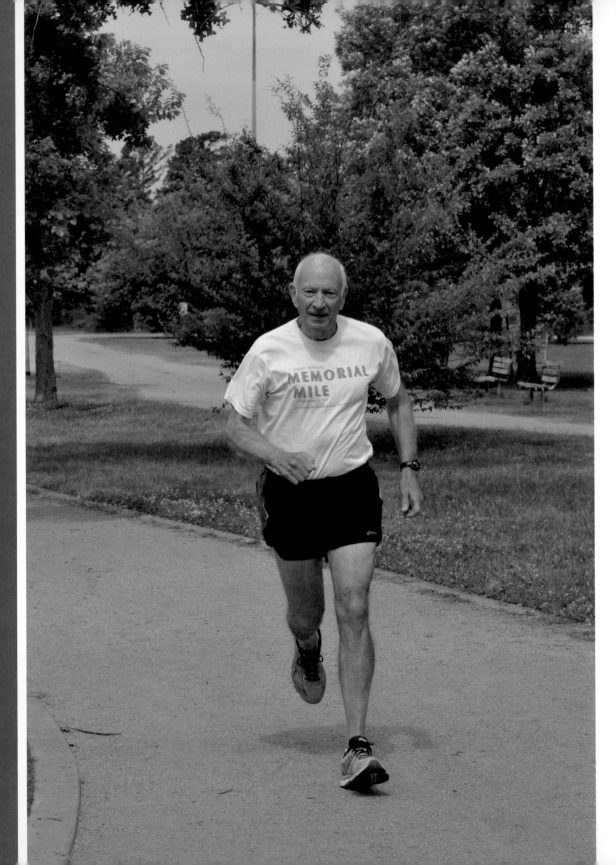

For me, the Park answers three basic, important needs: physical, social, and psychological. Once, when I climbed Mt. Kilimanjaro, I introduced myself to a man and told him I was from Houston. With envy and respect he replied, "You get to run at Memorial Park!"

TOWNES PRESSLER

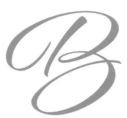efore going to Memorial Park, I started running at the Lamar High School track in 1978. My first day out, I wore a pair of tennis shoes with a collared polo shirt that was neatly tucked into my tennis shorts. I soon figured out that if I was going to be a runner, I needed different equipment. Also, after jogging a quarter mile, I knew that I had a lot of work ahead.

I finally ventured to Memorial Park in 1979. As I began to run more, it was wonderful to watch the weight come off, my body change, and my general health improve, but it was also interesting to be introduced to new words and expressions. At first, when my friends would ask if I was going to "do three," I did not know if they meant three miles, three loops, three minutes, or three-quarters of a mile. And then, what are a span, pick-up, interval, and hill work? There is an entire vocabulary that comes with running at the Park.

In the late 1980s, it was a big deal to be a part of the Houston Harriers running club, which was led by Coach Jim McLatchie. His basic philosophy for track workouts held that if we did not throw up by the end, we had not run hard enough and needed to do more. Before he would let me join the team, I had to submit a written paper regarding my experience, goals, and thoughts about running. I was excited when he finally reviewed my essay and allowed me to run with the Harriers.

Jim was an amazing coach. He was demanding and stretched every ounce of energy out of you at track workouts and in weekly schedules. He made a vast difference in many lives, including mine. He no longer lives in Houston, but occasionally we correspond, and I keep telling him how much I continue to appreciate and respect his coaching, leadership, and example, because I truly do.

Memorial Park has been quite a blessing to me, and there was a period of about fifteen years when it was my best friend. I was putting in 2,500 to 2,800 miles per year plus long days at work. I set my core priorities early, and one of my mantras was "I don't get paid to run." Obviously work came first, but running was a very close second. The folks dear to me did not understand my determination, and I ran so much that they thought I had lost my mind.

When social engagements conflicted with running at reasonable times, I adjusted. As soon as I got home, I would head to the Park to get in my miles, frequently between 11:00 p.m. and 1:00 a.m.

There were a number of times when I was at the Park in the early morning hours and saw people I knew, and it was just as if we had passed each other in the middle of the day. One of my favorite memories from running at such odd hours is of a man who was walking the loop and playing a trombone. It was a cool night with a light ground fog. The sound was beautiful, and the image was so peaceful and surreal. It is difficult to believe that could happen in the heart of a city of four million people. I am thankful that my wife, now, is a runner. She allows my friendship with the Park and understands the hours on the trail, but I do have to be careful to not let it dictate my life as it once did.

I also think the Park is extremely egalitarian. It does not matter where you went to school, what job you have, or where you grew up. Instead, the Park collects a cadre of people who are intensely interested in working hard. Everyone shows up in a shirt, shorts, socks, and shoes. They are judged only on their dedication to the sport and the effort they put in to reach their personal best.

The diversity seen throughout the City of Houston is also represented well at the Park, where various cultures are melded together. The Park's popularity and its circular trail remind me of the Latin American tradition of strolling around the town square with friends on Friday night. Because the trail is circular and three miles long, it's a very similar situation. It allows people to see and greet each other and is short enough that anyone can make it around.

For me, Memorial Park fills three basic, important needs: physical, social, and psychological. At my age, maintaining an active, healthy lifestyle is more important than it has ever been. The Park offers a great alternative to a gym or neighborhood running.

Socially, I have enjoyed teamwork and camaraderie while running on the trail and have developed lasting friendships. Runners not only have fun together, but through exercise, we are bonded together. It is a bonding not easily duplicated in a corporate setting.

Finally, Memorial Park is extremely therapeutic. It is a place to think things through, solve problems, and sort out priorities.

The Park is also home to many Olympic-caliber athletes such as Coach Al Lawrence, Sean Wade, Jon Warren, Joy Smith, Joe Flores, and on and on. As a middle-of-the-pack runner, I enjoy just getting to be a part of it all. There is a rush as the elites go flying by and leave me in their dust.

In 2015, I turned eighty. I have not been able to compete in a marathon for several years, but I am striving to run twenty-six miles—the length of a marathon—each week, with an occasional track workout. However, my body is pushing back on that quantity and intensity. I've recently dropped to an average of about twenty-two miles per week with some short pickups, but I am working to be able to run farther and faster again. The pursuit never ends!

Today I search for races in the Houston area that have an eighty-and-up age group, but most only go up to seventy-and-up. That is okay, though, because it keeps the pressure on. There are a few other men in their eighties who I have competed against for several years, and we are all still running hard. The eighty-and-up age group is extremely competitive, which is fun, but we also sincerely enjoy seeing each other do well.

I have traveled quite a bit and often find myself speaking to other runners from across the globe. Last year, midway up Mt. Kilimanjaro, I met a guy from Holland who, upon learning I was from Houston, commented, "You get to run in Memorial Park! I hope to do that someday." The Park is known the world over, and I am thankful to live in a city that has such a wonderful destination for runners and such a robust running community.

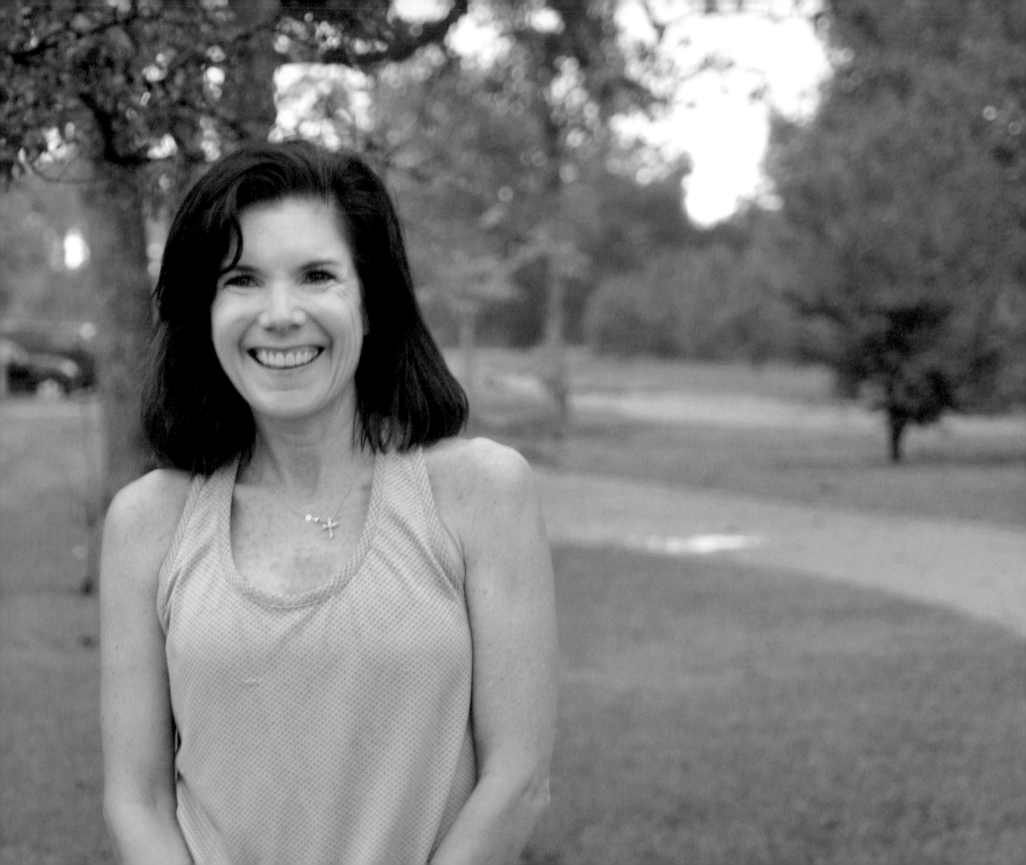

ROBIN PROCTOR

*I*n 1987, I read *I'm Running to Win* by Ann Kiemel. Although the book discussed the difficult experiences the author faced while training to qualify for the Boston Marathon, I was motivated and thought, *I can do that!* At that time there were not many women who were running marathons and definitely not many groups that trained on a regular basis. I bought *The Complete Book of Running* by Jim Fixx and followed the suggested schedules.

I completed my first marathon in January 1988 and will never forget the overwhelming feeling of crossing the finish line. That experience birthed a love for running that continues to this day. I worked out on my own until 1999, when I joined Kenyan Way, a newly formed group that provided training schedules and support during workouts. I met many wonderful friends, and we have continued to train together for the last seventeen years. We always meet at the Memorial Park Tennis Center. On days when we are struggling through the heat and humidity to complete a long run, we look to our running partners, the Park, and conversations along the trail to help us finish. We share our stories and lives with each other, which brings us together for more than just exercise.

I feel like the running community is very unique. There was a time when our training group included a wide array of individuals with many different backgrounds: anything from a construction worker all the way to a man who was the CEO of a large corporation. However, when we ran together, it did not matter. We all laughed together as we ran, regardless of our heritage and status. Running has always been a great equalizer.

When we all meet to work out, we do not consider our differences. Instead, we encourage each other, laugh together, and occasionally cry together. I am not aware of any other field or sport that is quite the same.

During the first seventeen years of my marriage, I had never been able to conceive. Shortly after I turned forty, I had an injury that prevented me from running so many miles, and to my surprise, I became pregnant. I continued to exercise up to the day my son was born, and the running community was with us every step of the way. Despite the fact that I lived in Clear Lake, which is thirty minutes away from the Park, I still made the daily drive just to be with my friends. I have fond memories of running at the Park while pregnant and anticipating the arrival of my son. He has been a tremendous blessing to my husband and me.

Five years after my son was born, I was diagnosed with breast cancer. I was shocked when I heard the diagnosis because I had worked so hard to maintain a healthy lifestyle. It was such a difficult time, but again, the running community was always with me. I went through a double mastectomy, chemotherapy, and seven weeks of radiation. There were times when I didn't feel well, but the minute I laced up my shoes, drove to the Park, and saw my friends, I always felt better. Today, I am a six-year survivor and attribute my healing to Christ, my family, and the running community. I treasure Memorial Park and the friends I have made over the last seventeen years. They are a significant part of my journey, and I am eternally grateful for them!

It is well to be up before daybreak, for such habits contribute to health, wealth, and wisdom.

ARISTOTLE

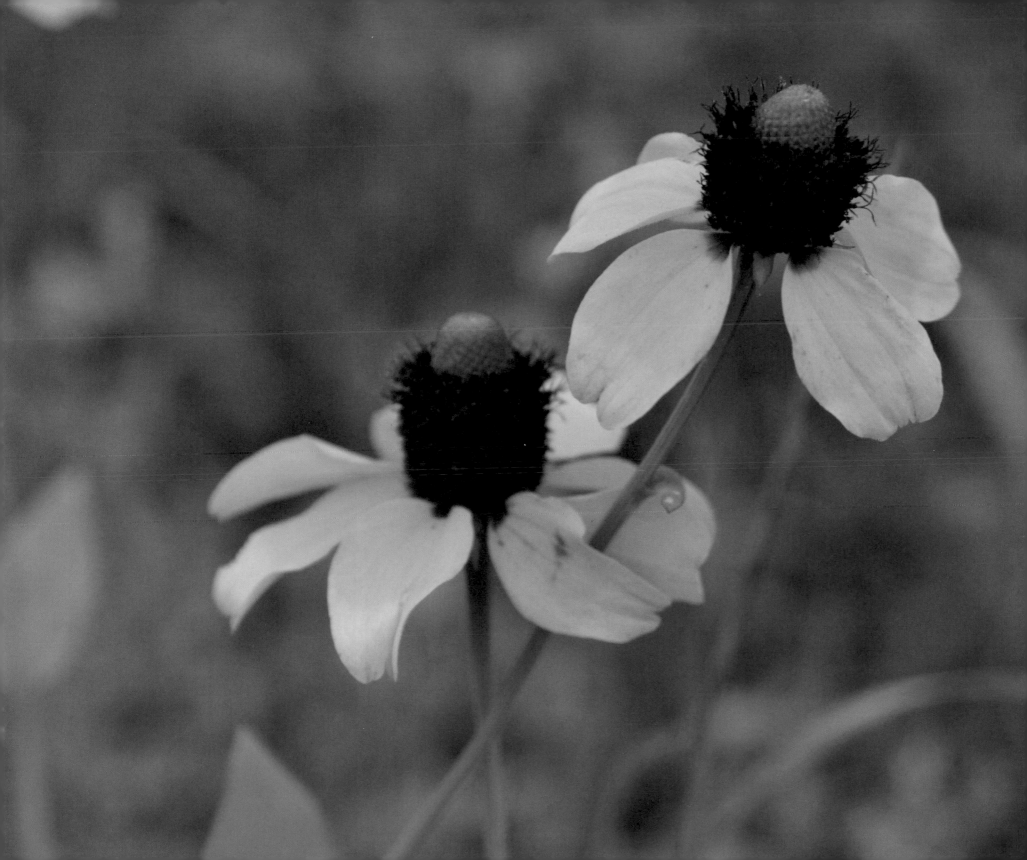

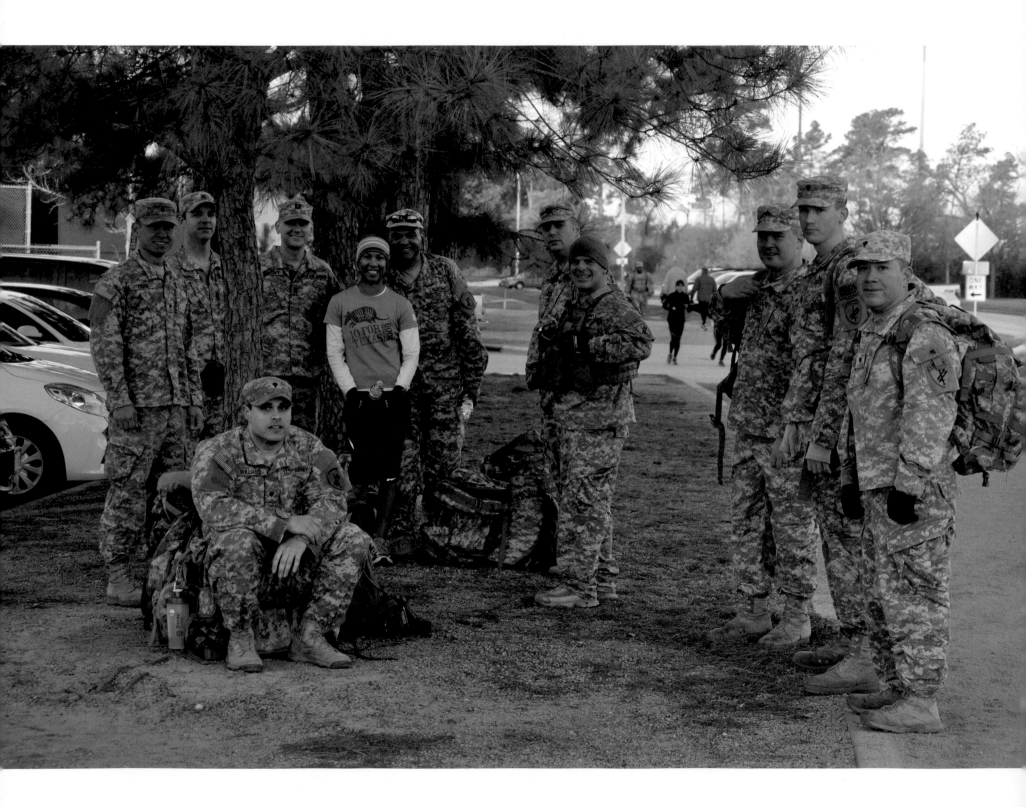

ARMY RANGER RESERVES

We meet once a month and are required to hike twelve miles while carrying at least thirty pounds in our backpacks. Occasionally we come to Memorial Park because it is centrally located and we enjoy being around the other people on the trail. We start at 3:00 a.m. so we can all finish by 7:00 a.m. and get back to our normal weekend activities. A few of us prefer to jog the entire way so we can get it over with as soon as possible. Once everyone is back at the Tennis Center, we get into formation and go over any business or plans that need to be discussed.

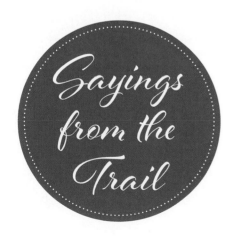

"I am going out long and coming in short."

The most popular place to start running is the Tennis Center. If someone is doing a longer run that leaves the Park, he can either do two miles and exit at one corner of the Park, or go the opposite direction and do one mile before leaving the trail. Going out long means you are doing two miles on the trail before leaving the Park. Going out short means you are doing one mile on the trail. The same is true when finishing a run: you can hit the Park and go straight back to the Tennis Center, which is a mile away, or go the long way around and get two miles in.

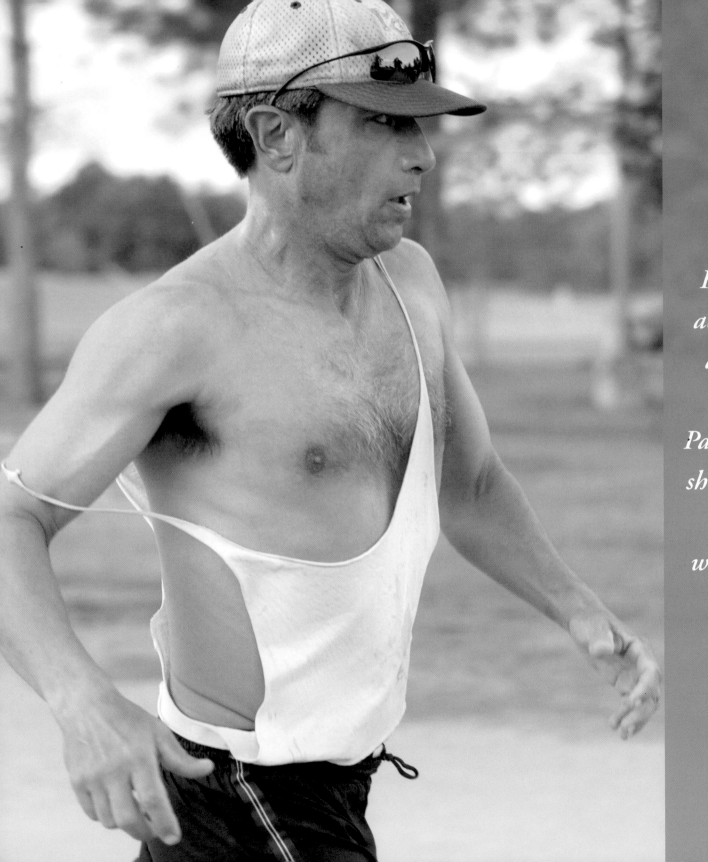

Few things in life are absolutely certain, but a couple of them are that I am not at the Park to put on a fashion show, and I do not have enough time to chat with all the nice people out there.

J. NOLAN RENOBATO

My parents raised me in a humble environment and instilled in me the importance of family and the value of working hard toward fulfilling my dreams and goals. I started playing organized baseball when I was five years old and have loved the sport ever since.

Throughout my playing career, many of the athletes I competed against were taller and heavier than me, but by the time I was eighteen, I was able to tilt the playing field in my favor. My natural speed and relentless determination earned respect from pro scouts. However, I opted to turn down a minor league contract offer in order to attend McNeese State University (MSU) in Lake Charles, Louisiana. This route was smartly chosen because my mother has always believed in the power of knowledge and encouraged higher education.

We had a great coach at McNeese who was strict and emphasized discipline through running and lifting weights. Our talent-laden baseball team could have won NCAA track meets or bodybuilding contests. After taking the Southland Conference Championship during the 1988 season, we ended in the top twenty-five after winning several games in the College World Series Midwest Regional tournament. Although an injury stymied any chance I had of getting into professional baseball after college, I learned many invaluable lessons participating in that program. I am truly blessed to have gained an unyielding belief in myself and a confidence in my athleticism. I also learned how to handle adversity and capitalize on opportunities. Today, I merely desire to properly represent the brotherhoods and institutions that conditioned my character because certain bonds that have been forged can never be broken or taken away.

During the last twenty-one years, I have accumulated nearly eighty thousand miles, with the vast majority of those logged at Memorial Park. Because of my success at the undergraduate level, I have never felt a need to prove myself through running. Oddly, I have never entered an "official" race, although there have been numerous times when I have completed nine or ten laps around the Park. For me personally, running allows time to sort out issues in my mind. It is a way to illustrate that each person is accountable to himself for carrying out his life's own empower-ments. Outside of cardiovascular health, I believe the greatest benefits of running are the accompanying physical pain and discomfort, which are real reminders that one is truly alive.

Many people at Memorial Park recognize me by the clothes I wear. I buy a plain white T and cut it up to match my custom style and comfort. I also wear solid black shorts, black socks, black shoes, and a MSU baseball cap. My routine is to wear my signature shirt until it gets too holey or a strap breaks. Sometimes a shirt wears out in a few months, but others have lasted a year or so. I usually wash my clothes after I run and feel like my uniform has become my own personal "brand." Like Albert Einstein, whose wardrobe did not change, its simplicity allows me not to worry about what I wear on the track. Even when I am dead tired, I can just seize my brand's label and get on with the business of running the Park.

There have been instances when people have offered me shirts or caps with their companies' logos. However, I am fiercely private and have declined to advertise for anyone else. Few things in life are absolutely certain, but a couple of them are that I am not at the Park to put on a fashion show, and I do not have enough time to chat with all the nice people out there. Rather, I am there to give my best efforts in demonstrating a positive example and establish a limitless standard of fitness.

I manage my own company, which has allowed me to remain firmly entrenched in my exercise regimen. Although I am best by far at arbitrage, government bureaucracies and large corporations have attempted to place restraints on my company's profitability. In fact, my professional experience in this line of commerce has led me to the Supreme Court of the United States. I pray that one day I will recover money owed to me from goliath corporate entities that claim they have been taken advantage of in business. Thus, another part of the reason I run is that I know preserving my longevity will permit me to never quit fighting toward the day when my cases are finally settled. I look forward to enjoying the benefits of my institutional-type trading strategy and to rightfully secure my life's due futures. Fortunately, through running, I am prepared to wage those wars until the day I die.

Today I live about thirty miles from the Park, but I am committed to train there on a regular basis because I am somewhat fixated on raising the bar in the community for a more health-conscious population. To me, the Park is like a tranquil sanctuary and spiritual place. I generally do not train with anyone, because I am able to find Zen in the midst of a run. I feel like I can unchain and release my soul from the earthly institutions that bind me, and I am truly thankful for the feeling liberty shares.

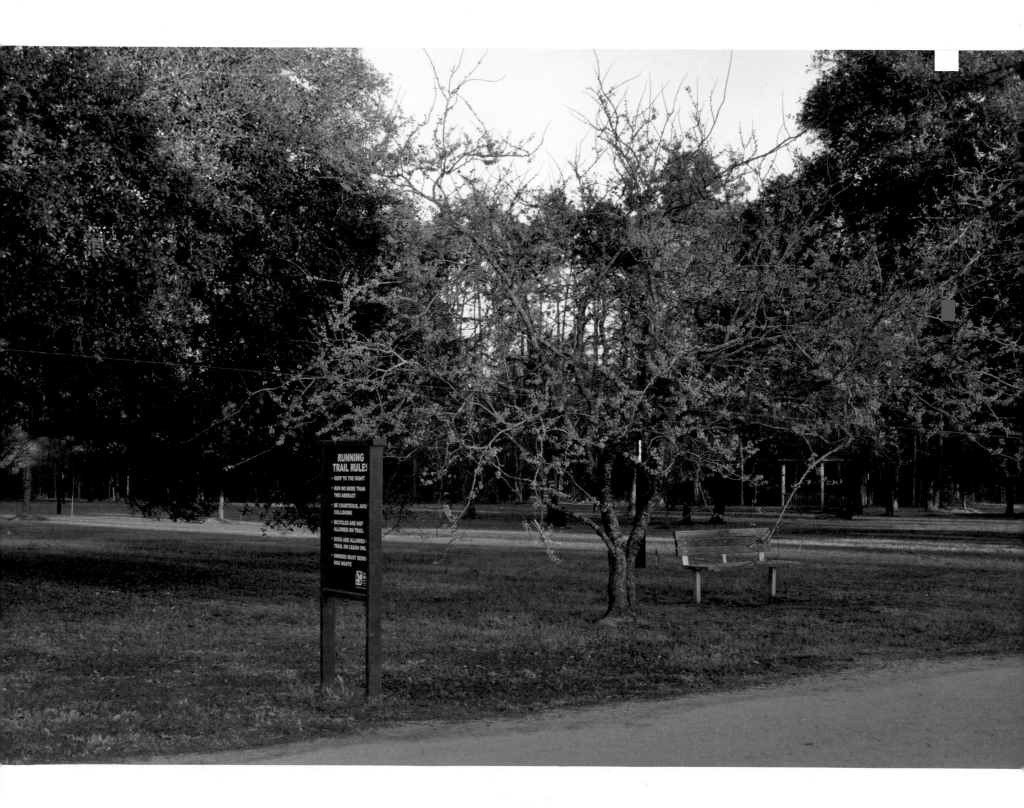

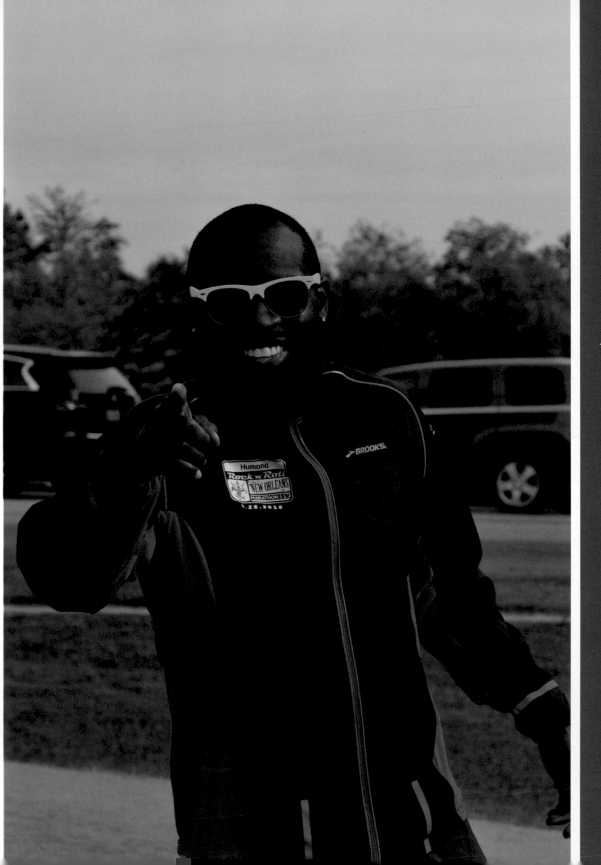

In 2013, after not exercising for five years, my coworkers invited me to go to the beach. As I was getting dressed, I had my "beach moment." I looked in the mirror and was in shock at what I had let happen to my body. The image of my stomach hanging over my shorts showed me that it was time to make a change.

EZRA RICHARDS

I was born in Trinidad and Tobago. When I was five years old, my mom brought my sister and me to New York City to get away from my dad. My mom has suffered from depression throughout her life, and we bounced around, living with friends and family for the next fifteen years. I started dancing as a young boy and by the time I was a teenager, I was performing in theaters throughout New York City.

During my sophomore year in high school, a friend suggested I join the track team. I knew I was fast but had never run anything more than a race down the street against my friends. I agreed to try running, but my life was extremely busy at that time. I would wake up at 6:00 a.m., do my homework on the train, sit in school all day, go to track practice, take a train to Manhattan and perform all evening, then try to get the rest of my homework finished on the train ride home at midnight. After four months of trying to maintain that schedule, I felt like I was losing my sanity.

One afternoon, as I was riding to dance practice, the train abruptly stopped and sat on the tracks for several minutes. The driver finally announced that we would not be going to Manhattan and were turning around. In the pit of my soul, I knew that was what I needed to do, too. I decided to quit dancing and focus on running. That was one of the best decisions of my life because I am still running today.

I received a scholarship to run track at Georgetown University, where I focused on the four hundred and eight hundred. In 2004, I qualified to run the four-by-four-hundred relay in the Olympics for Trinidad and Tobago. However, at the last minute I was told that I could not go, because the country did not have enough money to send me. Over the next few years, I continued to train and race the shorter distances. Occasionally I would throw in a seven-mile long run but not often.

Once, when I visited my family in Texas for Thanksgiving, I went out for a run but ended up getting lost. By the time I made it back to my aunt's house, I had done thirteen miles, and my legs felt like they had shards of glass in them. I had never felt anything like that before, and I hated it.

In 2007, I started grad school but was really struggling to maintain balance in my life. I would go from being full of energy to being so depressed that I could not get out of bed. I was finally diagnosed as bipolar and ended up being hospitalized. I moved back to New York City so I could get better and be close to my family. Unfortunately, I also stopped running, which was a bad decision.

After I started feeling better I took a job as a social worker, but it was not enough. Besides work, all I did was hang out with my friends, watch football, eat ribs, and drink beer. I felt like I wanted more in life and was frustrated at how lazy I had become. Then in 2013, after not exercising for five years, my coworkers invited me to go to the beach. As I was getting dressed, I had my "beach moment." I looked in the mirror and was in shock at what I had let happen to my body. The image of my stomach hanging over my shorts showed me that it was time to make a change.

A friend had just signed up for a half marathon, and she asked if I wanted to join her. At first I agonized over the memory of how terrible I felt when I got lost on my run in Texas. But I knew I needed to do something, so I agreed to start training.

A couple months later, I was jogging around Central Park, and it started snowing. People were looking out their windows watching the snowfall, but there I was, running . . . outside! The crazy thing was that Central Park was full of people who were doing the same thing I was. It hit me that must be the mentality of a runner. We are serious. Our attitude is, "Let's do this! Who cares about the weather?"

I was elated to finish the half marathon in the spring of 2014, but then I wondered, *What happens next? What do I do now?* The exercise had given me new direction, and I was finally feeling as though I was becoming my old, life-loving self. I decided to get certified as a personal trainer and finish my master's degree.

While in grad school, I joined a business fraternity and was elected president of my pledge class. I created a position called *director of health and fitness* and awarded points to members of the fraternity who exercised. I gave additional points if they worked out with a friend and had a prize for the person who accumulated the most points by the end of the year. As a result, we ended up having the healthiest pledge class in the history of the fraternity. I was so proud of the number of lives I saw change during that year. There were several members who began exercising for the first time in their lives, and most of them continue to work out today. I realized that I exude a culture of fitness. It is who I am as a person.

Once I finished grad school, I moved to Houston to be with my mom and help get her on the right track. She was still suffering from depression, so I decided to become her personal coach. I knew that if she would start eating healthy and working out, she would feel much better. Moving to Houston also gave me an opportunity to start from scratch. I wanted to make sure everything I did was about encouraging others, including my mom, to be healthy.

I started running at Memorial Park because a friend invited me. At first it reminded me of Central Park because I enjoyed being around all of the people, but I quickly realized there was one major difference. I felt like everyone in New York City was in their own world, but people at Memorial Park are much friendlier. I love how there is an entire area where people meet and socialize.

I continue to run at Memorial Park once or twice a week and finished my first full marathon in 2016. The only problem was I spent the whole race socializing. I kept meeting new people and talking to them. I am pretty sure I could have finished much sooner if I had just focused on running.

I feel like the whole world of distance running is new to me. I want to savor each race and appreciate how amazing it is that I am actually able to finish. I cannot imagine running a marathon every month like many people at Memorial Park do.

Before I moved to Houston, I had a few different jobs working nine to five. They were all claustrophobic to me. I could do the jobs, but I did not find happiness there. Instead, I have found satisfaction in working with people to help them become more healthy and active. I have no problem meeting a client at 6:00 a.m. for a workout. The funny thing is, there is no way I could have ever showed up for my office job at that time. Today, I am a track coach at a private school and a personal trainer. I love what I do.

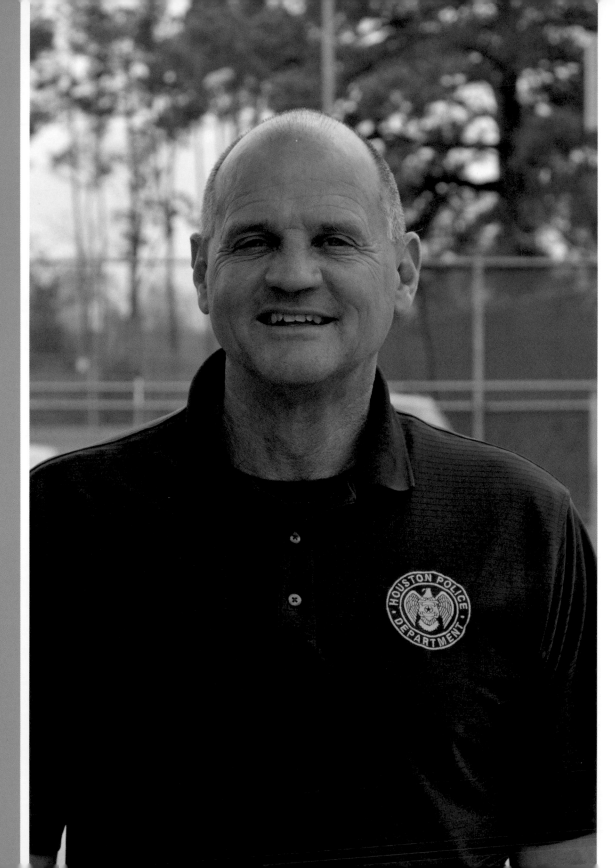

Many people see Memorial Park as a beautiful place where the only thing that happens is people work out, but that is not true. For the last thirty years, I have also seen the criminal side.

JAY ROBERTS

*I*became a Houston police officer in the early 1980s and was assigned to patrol Memorial Park. I was also assigned to work the Houston Marathon, and every year I would become inspired and insist that I was going to sign up the following year. After a while, it became the joke in my family because they knew exactly what I was going to say when I walked through the door after being at the marathon all morning.

Finally, after ten years of talking about entering the race, I decided it was time to commit. I finished my first marathon in four hours, nine minutes, but I was convinced that I could have broken four hours if I had pushed myself through the entire race. That was all it took for me to be hooked. I started really training hard and enjoyed working to get faster.

When I began running, my kids were attending a private junior high. I was asked to be the track coach, which I agreed to do during the four years they were at the school. It was fun to bring my sons to the Park because the other runners got to know them as well as they knew me. I was proud of their abilities and appreciated having them with me.

Many people see Memorial Park as a beautiful place where the only thing that happens is people work out, but that is not true. For the last thirty years, I have also seen the criminal side.

In the early 1980s, motorcycle gangs met on the south side of the Park. Shortly after we eliminated that problem, the Park became inundated with vast crowds on Sunday afternoons. Traffic would get so bad that it took an hour to get from Memorial Drive to the Tennis Center. Also, people were drinking and getting in fights. The officers who were stationed at the Park during that time grew frustrated, as it was not a safe place for every citizen.

In the early 1990s, the assistant police chief challenged me to come up with a plan to alleviate the problem. He said if it made sense, he would support it. We sectioned off one lane of traffic for police officers so they did not have to sit behind a mile of cars. Then we stationed plainclothes officers throughout the Park to identify underage individuals who were drinking. Finally, we put a paddy wagon on one corner of the Park and began arresting anyone who was breaking the law. The effort sent a message that we were serious about making the Park safe and enjoyable for everyone. It only took about six weeks for people to decide to go somewhere else because they were not having fun anymore.

During that same time period, we also saw an increase in public sexual activity on the south side of the Park. There were days when we would arrest twenty people for having sex in the bushes. We found out that we did not have to set up a sting to trap the individuals. They knew what they were looking for and just needed to find someone who was looking for the same thing.

We arrested a few men on multiple occasions. I do not always remember a person's name, but I can usually recognize a face. These men were so entranced that they did not even realize the same officer was about to arrest them for the third or fourth time. They would pull up in their vehicles, see the plainclothes officer sitting there, walk straight into the bushes, and take their clothes off. We started keeping statistics on the people we were arresting, and it was interesting to find out that a vast majority were married, upper-class men in their fifties.

One of the most frustrating things we still deal with on a regular basis is vehicle break-ins. Many of the individuals we arrest are repeat offenders. Burglary of a motor vehicle is a misdemeanor offense. Unfortunately, the city does not have enough jail space to house everyone convicted of a misdemeanor for an extended period of time. Most thieves are desperate and willing to risk a $250 fine if they can walk away with thousands of dollars of cash and items over time. They know and take advantage of the system. The Park is an easy place to find cars that are not locked or have valuables sitting in plain view. The thieves also know the vehicle owners are going to be gone for thirty to forty-five minutes.

I always tell people to use common sense. The best way to avoid a break-in is to not leave anything in their vehicles. It only takes a criminal seven seconds to see something valuable, break in, and be gone. It's also risky to put everything in the trunk. Even though a person's purse or wallet cannot be seen in the trunk, a thief can easily smash a window, hit a button to open the trunk, and then walk around to the back and take everything. Also, people at the Park should take their keys with them. All too often, they leave their keys resting on one of their tires or behind the gas cap, making them an easy target for those who happen to be watching.

When we start to see an increase in vehicle break-ins or any other problem, we target specific areas and work to catch the perpetrator. There is always at least one officer stationed at the Park, but many times, he is only backup for the undercover officers who are mixed in with everyone else. The people who use the trail would never realize that the person sitting on a bench, digging through a trash can, or jogging on the trail is actually a plainclothes officer looking for break-ins.

Sadly, Memorial Park is also a place where many people commit suicide. A majority of them have been on the south side of the Park, where there are dense trees and it is quiet. I do not know why the Park is a target for people who want to end their lives. I guess they think it is peaceful.

Today, I am a staff officer for special events in the City of Houston. Part of my job includes being a liaison between the Houston Police Department and the Houston Parks Department. The Memorial Park Conservancy and the Parks Department have really done a great job over the last few years. Even though they have half the manpower they once did, the Park looks better than it ever has. All in all, considering the number of people who use the Park, we have been fortunate there have not been more problems.

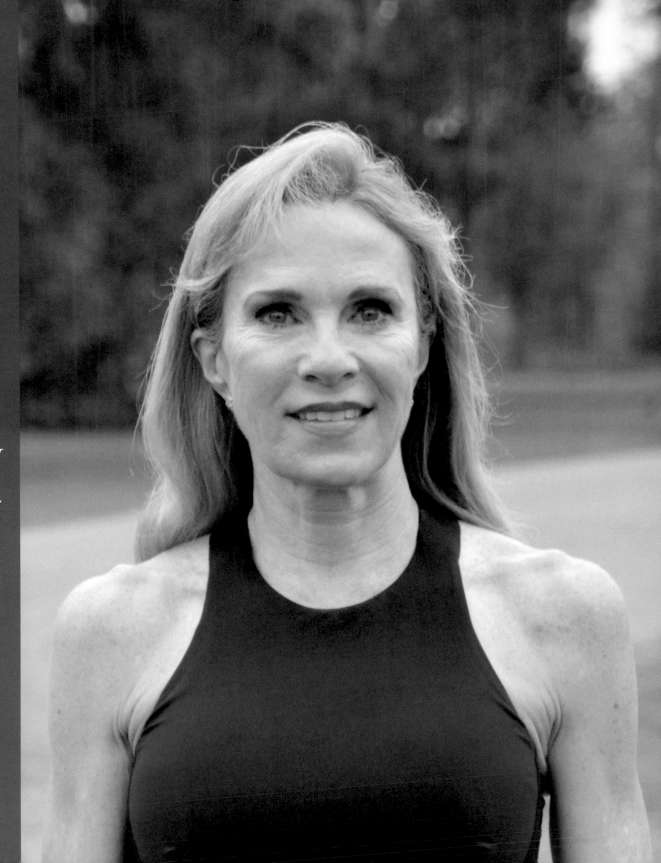

In 2011, at the age of fifty-two, I became the second woman to complete all fifty marathons in less than four hours each. Today I have run more sub-four-hour marathons than any other woman in the United States.

SUZY SEELEY

I have always maintained a healthy lifestyle. After my daughter and son were born, my workout regimen included running a couple miles a day for aerobic exercise. In 1995, I went to eat lunch with my son in his school cafeteria, never thinking it would change my life. I wore my workout clothes, and my son's teacher, Kristen Foxley, asked how far I usually ran. To my surprise, even though I was only running two miles each day, she encouraged me to start training for a marathon! I hesitated for a brief moment but promised I would make an effort to increase the distance of my run that weekend.

The following Saturday, on a warm August morning, I astonished myself by running five miles. It felt great! I became inspired to enter the upcoming Houston Marathon and ended up finishing the 26.2-mile race only four months after my inaugural five-mile run.

Kristen also invited me to accompany her to a Bible Study Fellowship meeting, and a few months later I became a Christian. When I look back at the tremendous influence she had in my life, I am thankful for the words of encouragement and sincere kindness she showed me. Although I have not run with or even seen her in many years, she is a fundamental part of who I am today.

I enjoyed my first marathon so much that I started entering races all over the country. Since 1996, I have completed 222 marathons and am ranked fortieth in the world for marathons completed by a female.

In 1997, I entered the San Francisco Marathon. Just before I left for the race, I read an article in the *Houston Chronicle* that suggested runners from Houston should get together in San Francisco. At that meeting, the newspaper columnist suggested I visit Memorial Park after I finished the race and returned to Houston. She insisted I would enjoy running with other people who were also training for marathons.

I decided to make the forty-minute drive to the Park and found a group of dedicated friends who enjoyed training as hard as I do. I also appreciated the softer surface of the Memorial Park trail. It has helped me to stay injury-free for most of my running career.

The people I train with originally started meeting at 6:00 a.m., but over the last fifteen years, our starting time has crept up to the point where a few of my friends have drawn the line. We start at 5:00 a.m. on the dot. If someone is late, he or she can catch us during the next loop. We are also strict about completing three miles on each lap. We generally run to the three-mile marker and then return to the Tennis Center for a drink of water. However, we do not count the jog back to the fountain as the beginning of the next lap. We stop our watches at three miles and then start again at zero because we like to be exact.

After I had finished thirty marathons, I started thinking that I should try to do one in every state. In 2011, at the age of fifty-two, I finished the Wineglass Marathon in Corning, New York, and became the second woman to complete all fifty marathons in less than four hours each. As of the summer of 2016, I have run 178 sub-four-hour marathons, more than any other woman in the United States.

I had actually completed fifty marathons in fifty states a few months prior to the Wineglass race, but my 1997 race in New York was not a sub-four. My daughter, Michelle, and I had entered the New York City Marathon, and unbeknownst to us, just before the race, her pancreas began shutting down. We had discussed that she had not been feeling well, but we did not know she had developed type 1 diabetes. I decided to stay with her during that race and am thankful I did. By the time we finished, she was vomiting, but in true Seeley fashion, she did not quit. It was worth extending the time it took to complete fifty marathons in less than four hours to be able to run with my daughter.

In 2013, some friends and I decided to join a tour group that offered to take us to a marathon in Antarctica and another in Chile a few days later. The only problem was that the weather in Antarctica was considered too dangerous for us to run, so the race organizers had to delay the start for a few days. Finally, the day came when we were supposed to run the marathon in Chile. However, we were still waiting for the weather in Antarctica to improve.

Just before we headed to the starting line of the race in Chile, we saw that the weather in Antarctica was finally beginning to clear. We joked that it would not be surprising if we had to journey to Antarctica as soon as we finished the race in South America. Sure enough, that is exactly what happened. I ended up starting the Antarctica race less than twenty-four hours after I finished the race in Chile.

After that trip, I decided that I should attempt to complete marathons on the other four continents so I could also join the "Conquering the Continents" club. I would also like to be able to say that I have accomplished a marathon on each continent in less than four hours. However, the conditions in Antarctica are less than ideal for running. I finished my 2013 race there in four hours, twenty-three minutes and tried again in 2015 but only ran a four-hour, twelve-minute time. The weather in 2015 was actually worse than it was in 2013. It was very difficult to run at all, much less maintain a sub-four-hour pace. I'll try again, God willing.

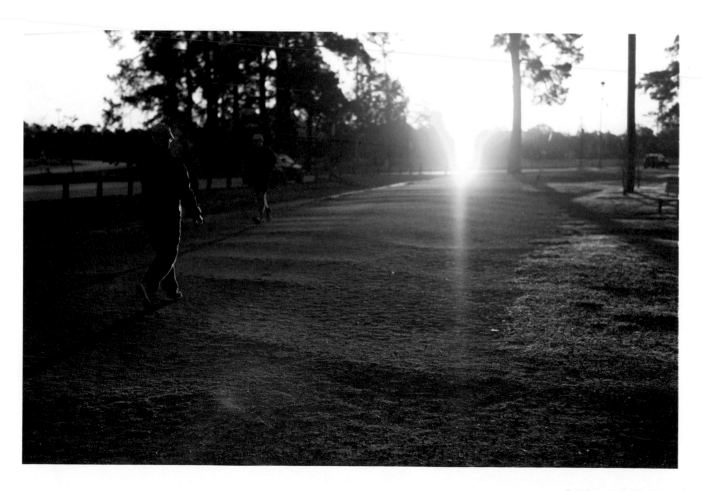

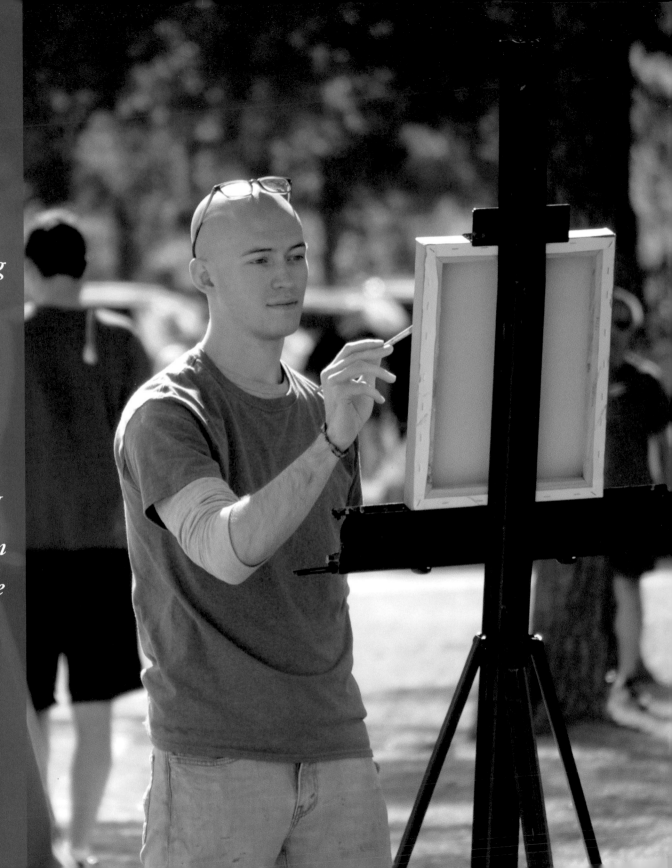

When I started painting full time, I did all of my work in the studio. But the studio became lonely, and cabin fever struck in the summer of 2015. Even though I would not call myself an extrovert, I do like to be around people.

ROGER SEWARD

I was born in Houston and graduated from Bellaire High School. I taught myself to draw as a kid and knew I wanted to become a professional artist, but I decided to pursue a degree in entrepreneurship from the University of Houston. I knew I could teach myself how to paint, but I needed someone else to teach me how to run a business.

I am known most for my paintings of fire hydrants, which I think are beautiful. As far as I know, no other artist in Houston is painting them. That is weird to me because they are so fascinating. I have yet to paint one of the new fire hydrants that were recently installed at Memorial Park, but they are also very appealing.

At the beginning of 2015, I also started noticing the vast contrasts in Houston's trees. There were many views that grabbed my attention because of the striking qualities of light. In the beginning, I did all my painting in the studio. But the studio became lonely, and cabin fever struck in the summer of 2015. Even though I would not call myself an extrovert, I do like to be around people. I also longed for windows so I could see the sunlight. After a couple attempts at taking my easel to the actual scene of the painting, I decided that I could still be somewhat productive even while working outdoors.

I am working to figure out the best way to adjust for the differences in painting in a still, quiet studio versus the ever-changing outdoor setting. Occasionally bugs land on my pallet, or a bird poops on my head. It's all worth it, though, because people are endlessly interesting, and the sunlight is refreshing.

I am also trying to overcome the wind, which occasionally sends my canvas tumbling to the ground. However, one benefit of painting outside is that the paint dries very quickly. When I am in the studio, the paint takes several minutes to dry, but when I am outside, it dries a few seconds after I put it on the canvas. This is helpful when I am ready to go home because I do not have to worry about wet paint in my car. I experimented with putting lights on my canvas so I could paint after the sun goes down, but the colors were too different, and I decided it was best to work with the natural lighting.

When I find a scene that grabs my attention, I usually take a photograph and then go back to my studio where I lay out the painting and organize my ideas. However, there are other times when I like the challenge of stumbling upon something interesting, setting up my easel, and starting to paint immediately. It is harder to start this way because I don't have a chance to plan everything, but I also think it is smart to practice that skill so I can get better.

Often I notice people creeping up as if they are scared to say something. Sometimes when I paint at Memorial Park, I've wished for an encouraging sign on my shirt that says, "You're not bothering me. You can talk to me!"

However, I do seem to be a magnet for people who need to vent. Most of the time their rants are rated PG, but there are a few individuals who are extremely inappropriate. Sometimes I will notice a person cozy up to me and can tell he is demanding eye contact. I am usually happy to stop painting and speak to him, but if I want him to go away, I just continue painting. He eventually gets the hint and leaves. I get invited to a lot of churches and am a target for people who want to enlighten me regarding their religious ideas.

One thing I have really enjoyed about being at the Park is letting kids help me paint. I happily lower the easel and hand them my brush. Sometimes they boldly insist they need a different color, which usually causes their parents to freak out. However, there is nothing that I cannot change or fix. Occasionally I am surprised at what they come up with, but more than anything, the experience gives them confidence and joy.

I also like to run at the Park because it is motivating. I usually run after the sun goes down and I have finished painting for the day. I do not like to get passed, which inspires me to run as hard as I can. I start rationalizing why that person is able to run faster than I am and tell myself he was not just standing on his feet, painting for three hours, which is obviously the only reason he is able to pass me. Then, it never fails that I realize I saw the same guy complete three or four laps around the Park *while* I was painting.

Recently I was having an introspective moment and realized that I was only painting for myself. Even though I expected people to buy my work, in the end, I was painting so I could get the idea out of my head and go to sleep at night. I decided to incorporate a selfless component into my work that would motivate me to paint more. Today, I pledge 10 percent of my sales to a charity that is relevant to each painting. When I sell a piece of art that depicts a scene at Memorial Park, for example, I make a donation to the Conservancy. Now, I am excited to sell something because it means I get to give something back. It feels good.

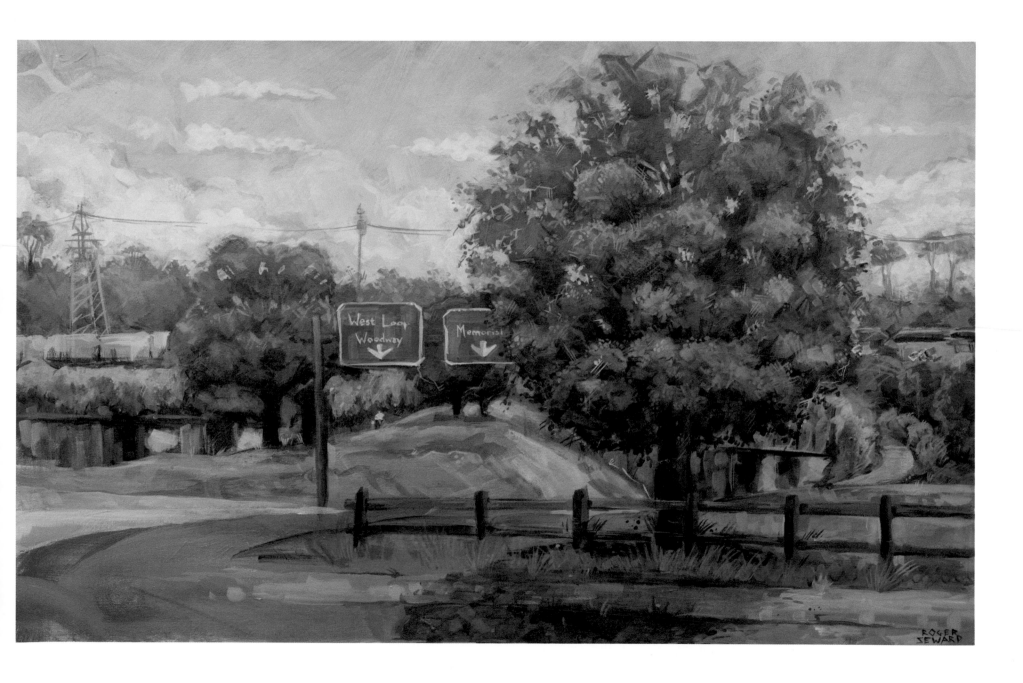

Regardless of whether I get out of my car with a blank canvas or am close to finishing a painting, people at Memorial Park are always so encouraging. As they run by, they often tell me it looks beautiful or they are glad I am capturing the beauty of the Park. Many people think painting at the Park is a hobby. When I tell them it is my full-time job, they are surprised. But Houston is a wonderful city for making a living as an artist. I think the city's diversity helps to bring appreciation and excitement, but there is also a rich history of Houstonians supporting their artists. Because of this tremendous support I have received during the last few years, I love being outside and making Houstonians' days just a little different from their normal routines.

A life becomes meaningful when one sees himself as an actor within the context of story.

GEORGE HOWARD

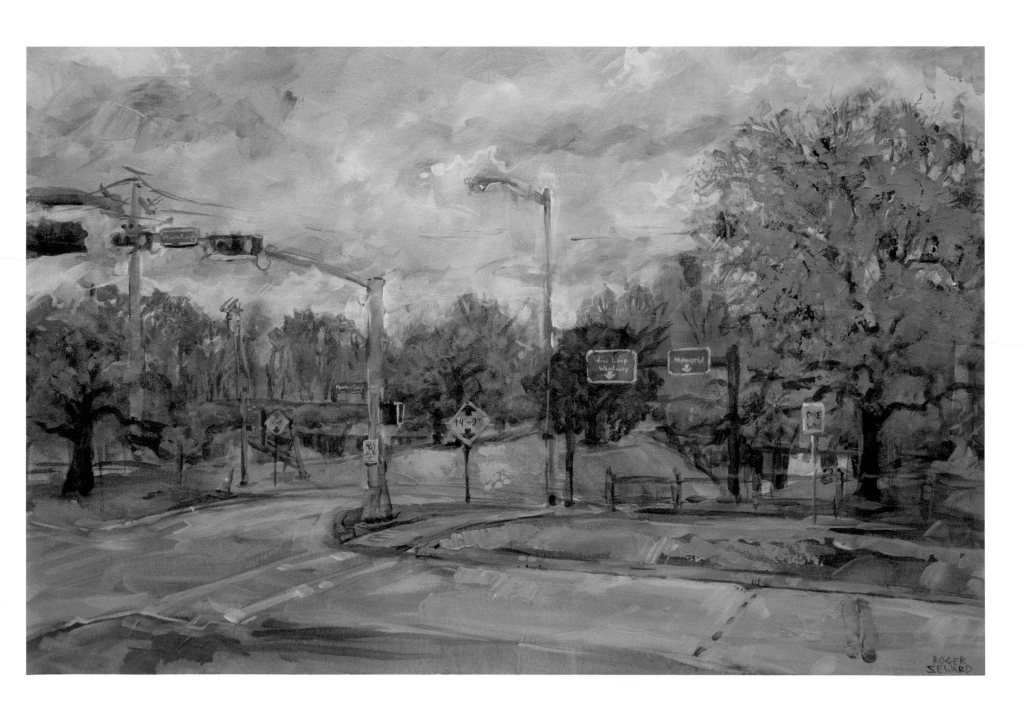

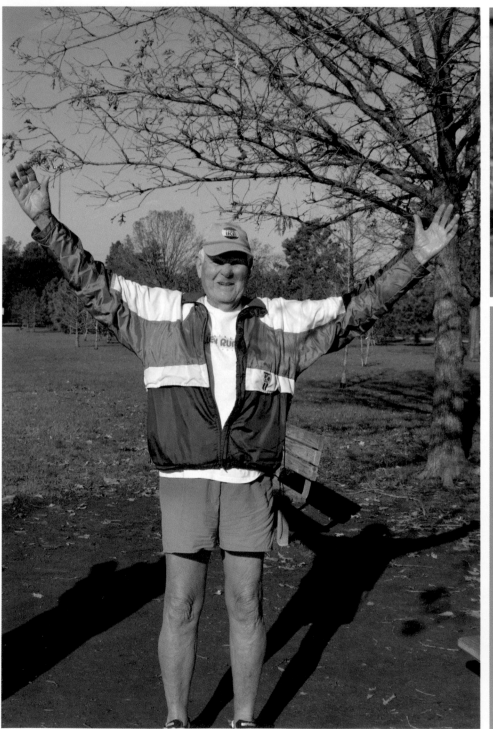

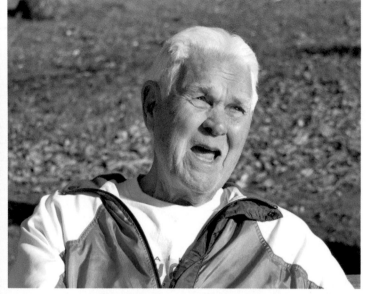

I like to set goals. In 2015, I did 168 miles but want to do better in 2016. I go to the Park three days a week and try to do at least four laps around the quarter-mile track. At the end of each lap, I raise my arms as if I have just won a race.

JOSEPH R. SHANNON, JR.

I grew up in the West Oaks neighborhood just beyond Memorial Park. In the late 1930s, my buddy and I rode our horses from my house and up Post Oak. Then we went across the only bridge that led to Memorial Drive and into the Park. There were only dirt trails then, but we would ride for miles through the dense trees and never see another soul.

I graduated from Lamar High School in 1942, just a few months after Japan bombed Pearl Harbor. As soon as I turned eighteen, I was drafted. I look back at that time when we were being trained to kill and handle unthinkable circumstances and realize I was only a child.

Over the years, many people have commented on my crystal-clear blue eyes. I have eighteen-twenty vision and only recently started wearing glasses to drive. However, I believe that my eyes are part of the reason I am alive today. When I was drafted, I was not allowed to enter the Air Force or the Marine Corps infantry, because I did not have twenty-twenty vision. A majority of the men I knew who joined the Air Force or infantry were killed during the war.

Instead, I was enlisted in a new division that was being developed called the Naval Combat Demolition Unit (NCDU), one of the precursors of the Navy SEALs. Although I was never deployed, I was in tremendous physical shape and confident that I could endure any conditions the war may bring. We spent many, many hours learning how to survive in the water. On several occasions, we were dropped off in the middle of the ocean and forced to tread water for ten or eleven hours before we were finally picked up again. Some people think those experiences would cause me to never want to be in water again. Instead, after I left the Navy, I continued to swim to stay in shape. I still enjoy swimming at the Houston Racquet Club a couple times per week; I just don't spend half my day there.

During World War II, the government gave us a stipend to buy cigarettes. As a young kid who was glad to see the sunrise each morning, the idea that smoking would kill me twenty years later was meaningless. I lived for the moment. So when some old, fat doctor told me smoking would cut my wind and might even be bad for my lungs, I could have cared less!

My assignment with the NCDU ended shortly after I turned twenty-one. By the time I got out, I was hooked on tobacco. Over the years, I would quit for six months or so, but I always eventually picked the habit back up. My wife started the running stuff. In 1973, Stratford High School was built across the street from my house. We began running on their track, but I continued to smoke. I was finally able to quit smoking when we joined Al Lawrence's group at the Memorial Park track in 1987.

I started a dozen marathons but only finished about half of them because something would happen. My wife and I are very competitive. When we were younger, we would run to the Park and back from our home, which was an eleven-mile round trip. We never actually ran together, though. Any time we were running at the same time, it was always a race. She never let me beat her and was usually a couple blocks ahead of me by the time we finished. I could never keep up with her. Her best marathon is ten minutes better than mine. However, I am proud of her. She was an age-group winner of the Houston Marathon, something I could never even dream of being.

I like to set goals. In 2015, I did 168 miles but want to do better in 2016. I go to the Park three days a week and try to do at least four laps around the quarter-mile track. Occasionally, when I have time and feel good, I do five laps. I jog the straightaways and walk the curves. At the end of each lap, I raise my arms as if I have just won a race. Then I sit down on the bench to catch my breath and talk to Al or anyone else who stops by. As soon as I am ready again, I get back up and do another lap.

When I turned eighty, I threw myself a big party at the Houston Racquet Club. The only thing I did for my ninetieth birthday was dive off the high dive there. A couple minutes later, my great-granddaughter jumped off. Then her dad, my grandson, decided he needed to dive off so he wouldn't be humiliated by his daughter and grandfather.

I've been happily married for forty-six years but am not ashamed to admit that I come to the Park to look at all the pretty girls. A few years ago, a van from a local radio station was out at the Park. They came up and asked if they could interview me. A couple minutes into the interview, the guy asked what keeps me young. I told him, "I am not young, but the two things I enjoy in life are old whiskey and the young women at the Park." It does not matter how old a man gets, he cannot deny that the view from the bench at the Memorial Park track is superb!

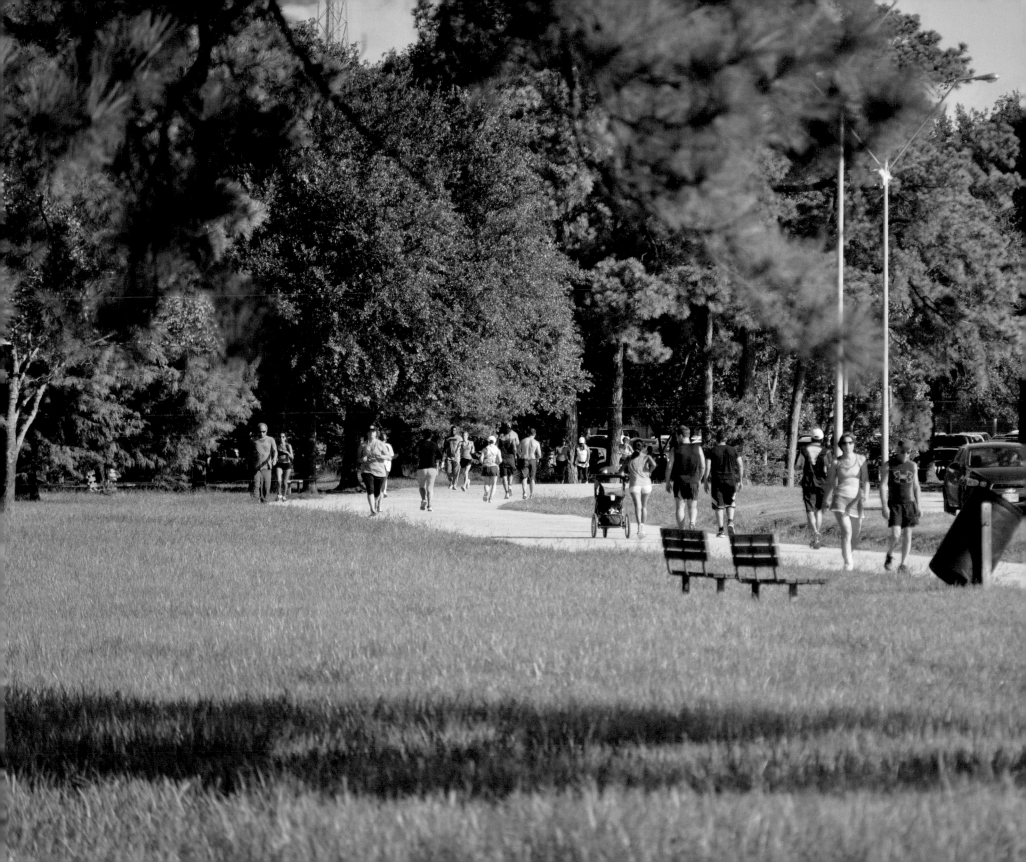

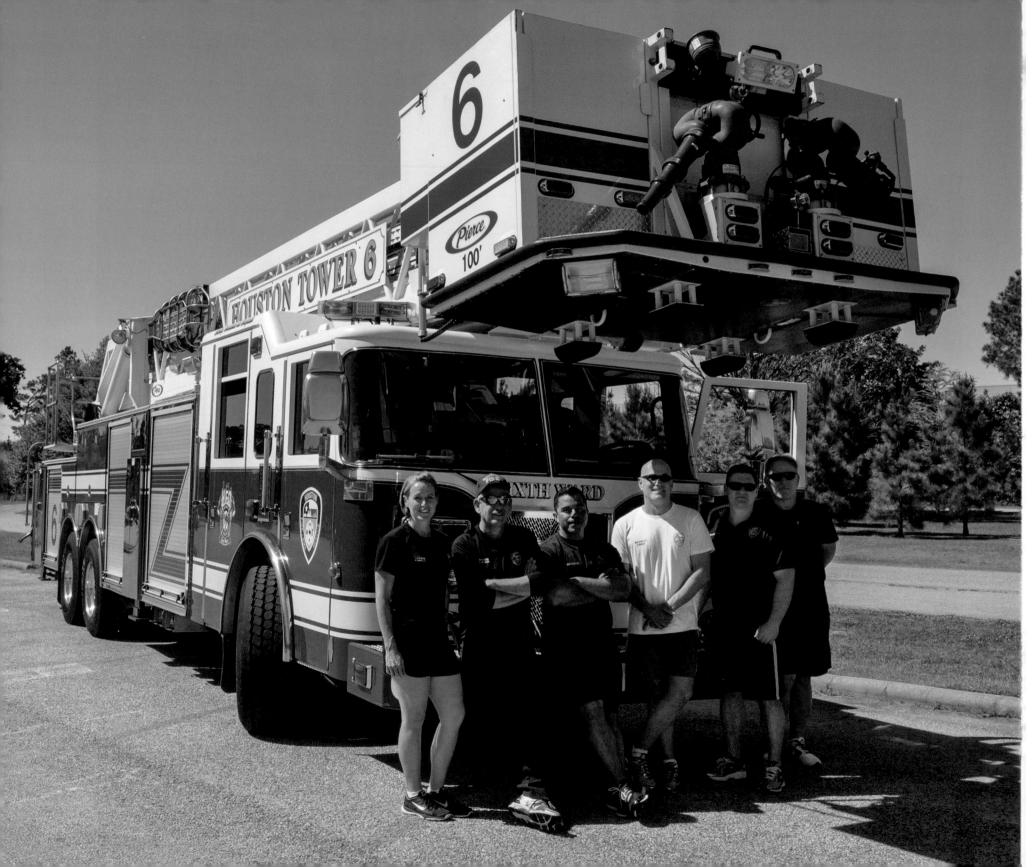

STATION 6, B SHIFT

Station 6 is on Washington Avenue, just east of Heights Boulevard. We take running and weight training seriously on the B shift. One of our firefighters, Andrew, tracks each person's progress and effort. He makes sure we find time to work out, and we try to get out to the Park once or twice a week. If a call comes in, we have to be back at our truck in less than sixty seconds. A few of us walk the quarter-mile track and stay close to the vehicles while the others run the trail. We enjoy getting away from the station for a few minutes, but our main priority is to stay conditioned so we can protect the people of Houston.

I do not know for sure if running has added years to my life, but I do know that running has added life to my years.

AL LAWRENCE

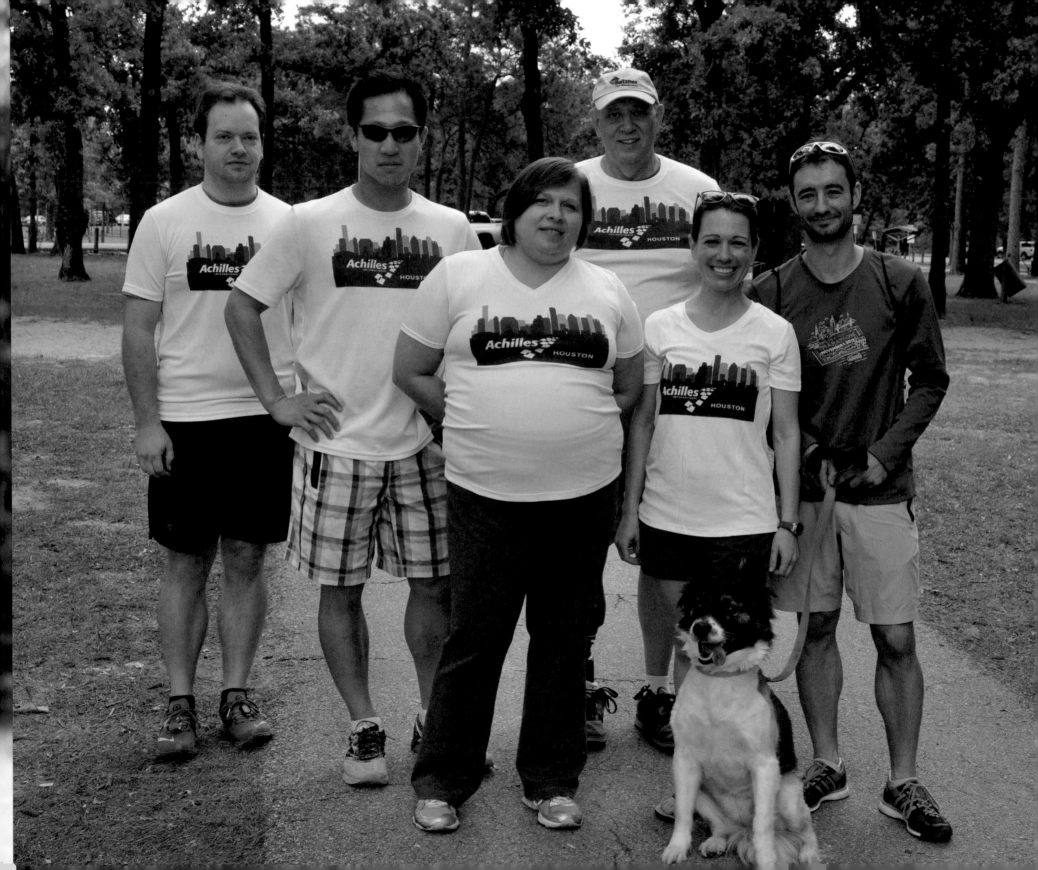

BERNIE TRETTA & ACHILLES INTERNATIONAL

The Achilles International organization helps disabled persons participate in sports and remain active. We started the Houston chapter in 2013 and meet at Memorial Park every Saturday. Before we head to the trail, we pair an able-bodied volunteer with each athlete to offer support and encouragement. We also plan exciting, unique events throughout Houston. Many of them involve drinking beer during or after the event.

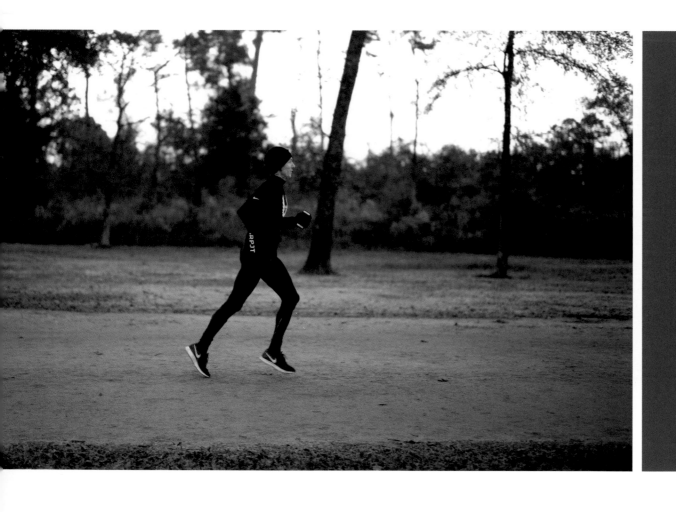

*There was a week in 1996
when I was training for the
Olympic marathon and did
forty-two laps around the Park.*

SEAN WADE

I run at Memorial Park almost every day because it is close to my home, and the trail's softer surface helps prevent injuries. There was a week in 1996 when I was training for the Olympic marathon and did forty-two laps around the Park.

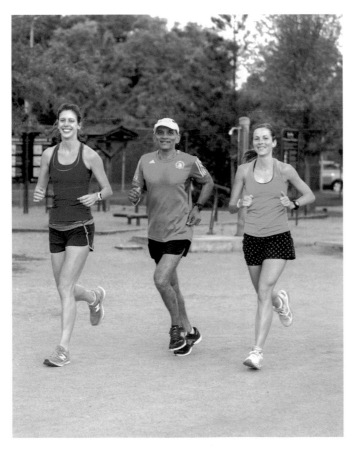

You cannot propel yourself forward by patting yourself on the back.

STEVE PREFONTAINE

As soon as I graduated from high school, I joined the Navy and worked as a machinist on an aircraft carrier off the coast of Vietnam. When I got out of the service, I found myself going through the same struggles I had watched my parents experience. I realized that I did not like who I had become and was desperate to find myself. I even tried to commit suicide several times. I was sent to prison just after I turned twenty for armed robbery, but I was actually glad to finally be punished for all the bad things I had done.

After I got out of prison, I married my high school sweetheart, but I was still too busy chasing women, doing drugs, and drinking. I didn't understand what a true man was really about, and I was arrested again. At the trial, my entire family came to the sentencing phase to try and convince the judge I was a good person. However, the judge told my family he wanted to make an example out of me and promptly sent me back to prison.

While I was in prison the second time, I received a picture of my wife, who was pregnant with our son. It was the most beautiful thing I had ever seen! Suddenly I found myself desperately wanting to be free.

Then, shortly before I was released on parole, I had a spiritual awakening and felt like I was going to explode with energy. I lay in my bed all night staring at a bright light and never went to sleep. The next day I decided that I needed to start reading books, newspapers, magazines, or anything I could get my hands on. A prison chaplain gave me a Bible, and I read it so much that I finally had to ask for another one.

Sadly, upon entering the free world again, I found myself locked into doing the same terrible things I had done before. My first marriage ended in divorce, and I was quickly remarried and divorced for a second time. I finally made a decision that if I really wanted to give up my bad habits and turn my life around, I had to do it for Jesus Christ's sake and not my own. When I was married, I tried to insist that my wives needed to change their behavior. Now I realize that I was the one with the problems, not them. I have also learned to believe in myself and have patience.

I love my life today. I have learned there will be ups and downs, but what matters is how I deal with them. I believe everyone can truly find their purpose if they look in the right place.

I want to change my name to "Wind Fork," because it represents who I have become. I am the Wind, which is carried throughout the world to spread good news or life-sustaining food. However, even though I can point people in the right direction to find the truth, I cannot force them to accept, or eat, what I give them. They must be willing to pick up the Fork and make the necessary changes on their own.

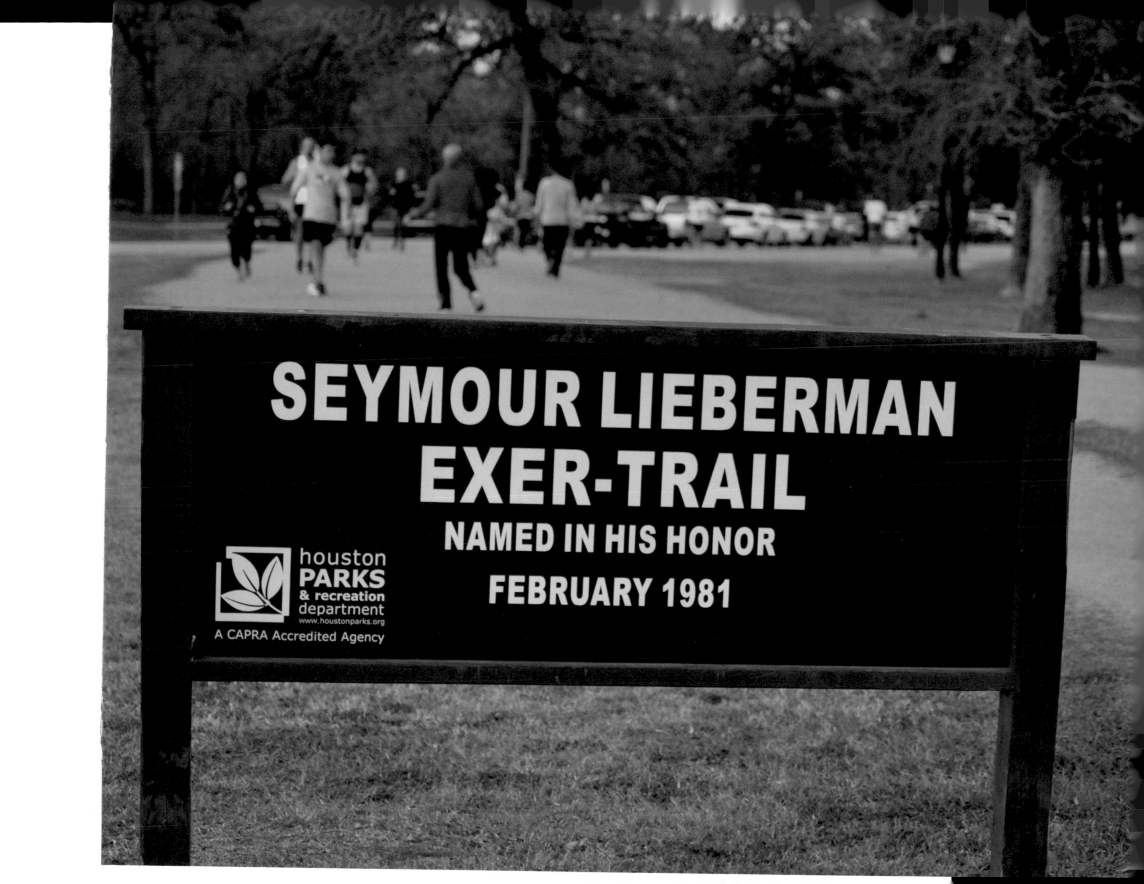

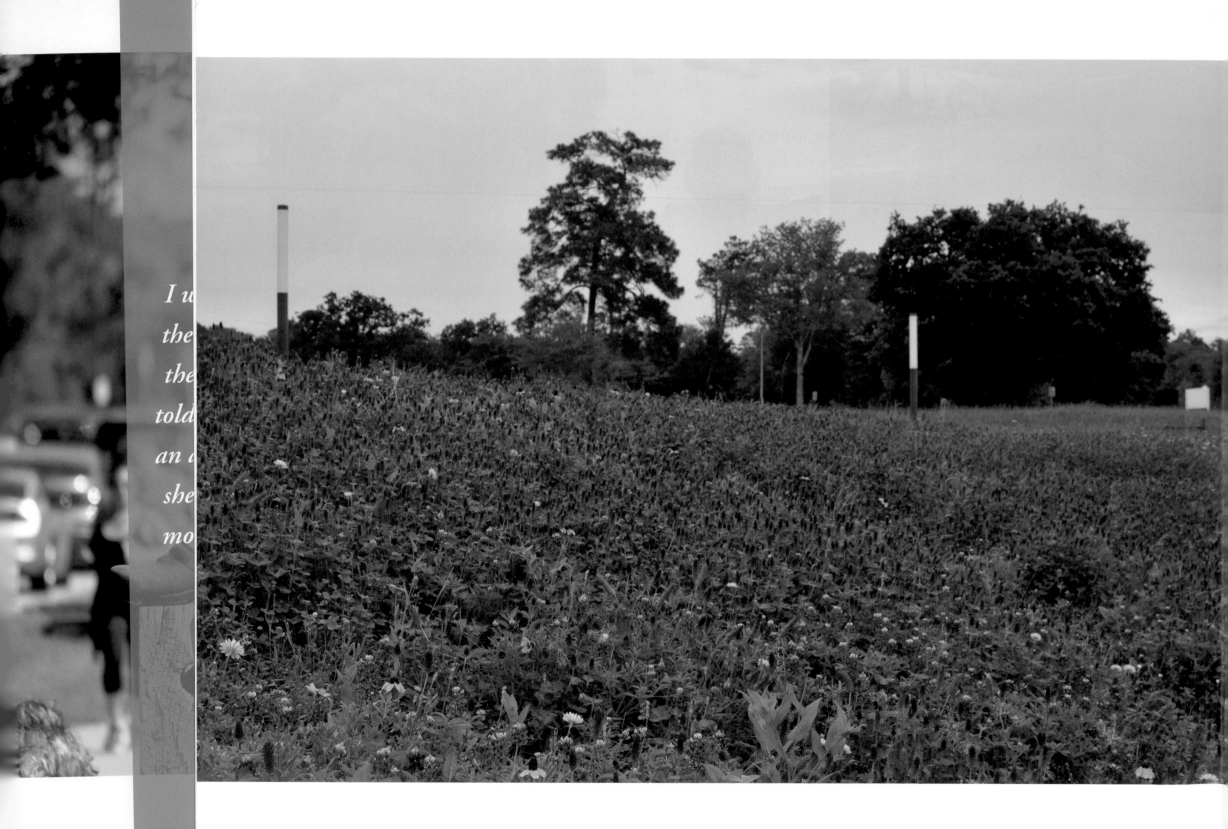

I w
the
the
told
an
she
mo

Photo Credits

George Bush Presidential Library and Museum – 22, 23

Candice Corley – i, 6, 8, 10, 12, 14, 18, 24, 34, 44, 58, 70, 72, 78, 84, 92, 96, 99, 106, 110, 114, 124, 140, 144, 159 (top right), 160, and 162 (top right)

Wilmer Gaviria – x (right), 53, 82, 87, 142, 159 (top middle and bottom right), 162 (bottom right), front jacket flap (bottom)

Brin Graham – 157 (top)

Pamela Hamza – 157 (bottom)

Kate Holden – 50, 81, and 143

Mark Holden – x (left) xiv, 2, 41, 42, 69, 127, 135, 147, 162 (bottom left), back cover, and front cover (bottom right)

Stacy Holden – 28, 32, 48, 66, 88, 100, 105, 128, 130, 132, 159 (top left and bottom middle)

Zachary Nottingham – 38, 54, 62, 75, 76, 102, 118, 136, 148, 159 (bottom left), 162 (top left), and front cover (top middle)

Richard "Austin" Pett – 129

Lance Phegley – 152, 156 (top)

Roger Seward – 121 (*Sunny Day at Memorial Park*), 123 (*Grey Day at Memorial Park*)

Ken Maurice Kellogg – 156 (bottom)

Chris Wenz – 158

Eric Youmans – xiii

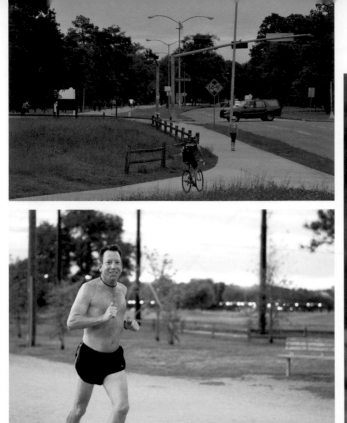
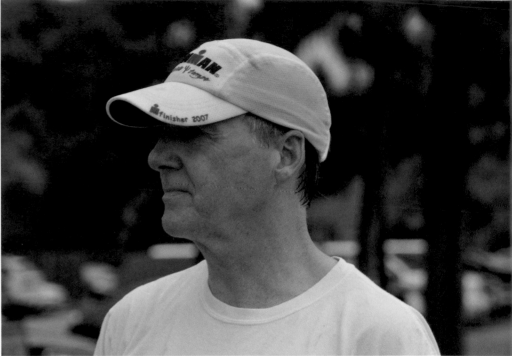
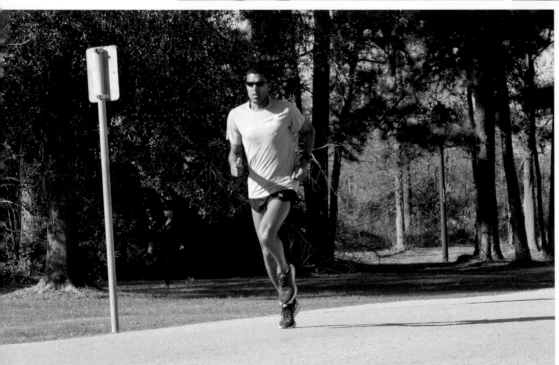
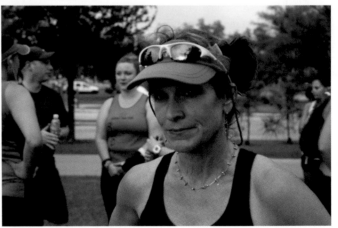
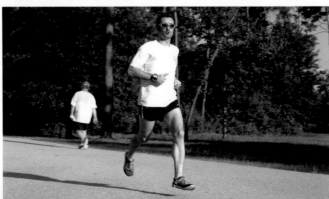